I0589377

Water Must Flow Uphill

Water Must Flow Uphill
Adventures in University Administration

Roger Makanjuola

AMVPS

AMV Publishing Services
P.O. Box 661
Princeton NJ 08542-0661
Tel(s): 609-5770905 & 732-6476721 Fax: 609-7164770
e-mail: publisher@amvpublishingservices.com
world wide web: www.amvpublishingservices.com

Water Must Flow Uphill Adventures in University Administration
US/International Edition
Copyright © 2013 Roger Makanjuola

First published in Nigeria in 2012 by
Mosuro Publishers
5 Oluware Obasa Street, Bodija
P.O. Box 30201
Ibadan Nigeria

All rights reserved. No part of this publication may be reproduced, stored in a retrieval system, or transmitted in any form or by any means, electronic, mechanical, photocopying, recording or otherwise without the written permission of the Publisher.

Book and Cover Production: AMVPS based on
Original Book Design by Festus Agboola and
Original Cover Design by Biodun Adeogun
Cover Photo Credit: Kolade Mosuro
Cover Re-origination: Ify Anyanwu
Cover Finishing: Dapo Ojo-Ade

Library of Congress Control Number: 2012916314

ISBNs: ISBNs: 0-9766941-8-2 (10-digit) --- 978-0-9766941-8-2 (13-digit)

Contents

Preface

They say every person has a book in him. This is mine.

The book covers a major part of my working life; the period when I was the Chief Executive of the Teaching Hospital at Ile-Ife, Nigeria, and then the period when I was the Vice-Chancellor of the University in the same town. It is not a description of administration per se, but of my personal experiences during the time. It took me four years to write, because I did the typing myself and I was engaged in my normal responsibilities as a consultant psychiatrist and lecturer throughout the period.

The book includes many harrowing tales as well as happier times. However, this is essentially an account of the love I have for Great Ife—the hospital as well as the University. It is a love story; a tale of true love. Readers may well ask how a person can be expressing love of a physical entity. Any person who has lived and worked in our beautiful campus and unique hospital will easily understand. As for those readers who have not had that privilege, after they have read this account, perhaps they also will understand.

GREAT IFE!

Roger Makanjuola
Ife, 2012

Acknowledgments

I wish to thank the following individuals without whom this book would not have been possible.

A number of individuals provided essential information or assistance in cross checking the accuracy of some information. These included Professor Biodun Adediran, Mr. Nick Igbokwe, Dr. Bola Mapayi, Professor Femi Ajibola, Mr. Victor Ado and Professor David Ijalaye. The Registrar of the University, Mr. Ayo Ogunruku, kindly permitted me to go through the records of the University Council and Senate, and Mrs. Dorothy Salami and Mrs. Dorrit Ocan facilitated the examination of these records. My wife, Dorothy, encouraged me to make this record for posterity and to keep on until it was completed.

Finally, I must thank the publisher, Kolade Mosuro, for going through the manuscript, seeing value in it and then putting in the painstaking editorial work. My friend, Professor Akin Aboderin, was the one who suggested that I submit the work to Kolade; I am indebted to him for this.

Dedication

This book is dedicated to the delights of my life, my grandchildren—Mia, Elena, Mekhi, Alicia, Micah and Tiago.

I

My Baptism into Administration

I was sitting in my office with the Director of Administration (DA) and the Assistant Director in charge of general administration. We had just returned from a visit to the Wesley Guild Hospital, one of the four hospital units of the Ife University Teaching Hospitals Complex. We were all tired after a long and rigorous tour around the hospital on a very sunny day—this was late in July 1985. We were dealing with the final task of the day which was sorting out applications for vehicle loans. We were quite preoccupied with this rather boring task when the Director's secretary came in and whispered to him. They both went out, and a minute later the Director came back in and said there was "something in the news" about the appointment of a new Chief Medical Director (CMD). I asked him who it was; he replied that he didn't get the name. I left him and went into his office and asked his secretary who had been appointed as CMD. He answered, "It is Professor G.O.A. Ladipo." Professor Ladipo was then the Director of Clinical Services of the institution. I tidied up the files on my table and went home.

I had been appointed Acting Chief Medical Director of the Ife University Teaching Hospitals Complex ten months earlier in August 1984 following a major crisis in the institution. That crisis will certainly go down as a turning point in the history of health services in Nigeria in view of the major effects it had on the teaching hospital system. The origins of the crisis are best understood in the context of the history of hospital administration in the country.

Initially, the administration of government hospitals lay firmly in the hands of doctors. The Medical Superintendent, always a doctor, was the unchallenged boss of the hospital, in spite of the fact that he had no training in management whatsoever. However, the system appeared to work fairly well. The exception was with the teaching hospitals. Right from its inception, the University College Hospital (UCH), Ibadan had a House Governor rather than a Medical Superintendent, the forerunner of the Director of Administration. This concept was adopted by the Lagos University Teaching Hospital (LUTH) when that institution was founded, but the scope of authority of the LUTH Hospital Administrator was somehow reduced by the fact that LUTH was, at least in theory, under the supervision of the College of Medicine.

In the University College Hospital, the House Governor reigned supreme. One of the best known was Colonel J.B. Robertson, a retired British army officer, who held the post in the 1960s. His word was law. He was not a medical doctor, and I am fairly sure he was not actually a trained hospital administrator. However, under him UCH was managed admirably well. Subsequently, the term House Governor was changed to Director of Administration, and the Director of Administration continued to be in charge. The system was adopted by other teaching hospitals as they came into being.

In the 1970s, things started to go wrong. There was increased dissatisfaction with the system. The reasons probably included political and professional considerations, as well as, possibly, deficiencies in the professional performance of some of the hospital administrators. The reasons raised here are mere speculations. In any event, there is no doubt that there was much dissatisfaction with the system and members of the medical profession were among the most dissatisfied. The complaints became louder and louder, and got to the ears of the Federal Military Government. Anecdotal information has it that a senior doctor who was close to the then Head of State, General Olusegun Obasanjo, whispered into his ears about how badly the teaching hospitals were being run, advising him to take drastic action to resolve the problem.

In an attempt to resolve the matter, the Obasanjo-led Federal Military Government issued Decree Number 74 in 1979. This Decree made the Deans or Provosts of the associated medical schools responsible for the administration of teaching hospitals and designated them as Chief Medical Directors. The Director of Administration was to be responsible to the Chief Medical Director. This move was acclaimed by the medical and other health professionals. However, there were drawbacks. The new Chief Medical Directors were already fully occupied in their capacities as Provosts and Deans. In reality, their second appointments as Chief Medical Directors were part-time ones. It was, therefore, very difficult, if not impossible, for them to manage the affairs of their teaching hospitals effectively or to exert their authority. Some Directors of Administration took advantage of this to remain effectively in charge.

In 1983, there was a crisis at the Ife University Teaching Hospitals Complex, where there had been a long standing conflict between "administrators" and health professionals—not just doctors. One of the major issues was the tussle between the Chief Medical Director and the Director of Administration for control of the hospital. The crisis resulted in a violent strike action which led to the closure of the institution for virtually one year. At the height of the crisis, there was an invasion of one of the hospital units by Mobile Policemen who were furious over the perceived failure of the hospital to treat one of their colleagues. One of the findings of the Umaru Shehu Administrative Panel of Enquiry which looked into the case was that the system involving a dual role for the Provost/Dean as Chief Medical Director was unworkable. The Panel's recommendations resulted in Decree No. 10 of 1985 (now Cap. U15 of the Laws of the Federation of Nigeria, 2004). This decree provided for a full-time Chief Medical Director (CMD) who was clearly defined as Chief Executive. Decree 10 is still in force. The current administrative structure of teaching hospitals is based on the contents of that decree.

The Government accepted the Umaru Shehu panel's recommendation that, pending the appointment of a substantive Chief Medical Director, it should appoint an Acting CMD from among the academic medical staff of the Faculty of Health Sciences of the University of Ife, acting on the advice of the Vice Chancellor (VC). The VC, Professor 'Wande Abimbola, recommended me for the appointment. There was widespread criticism of his choice, but he stood his ground and eventually, on a morning in August 1984, I got the letter of appointment. I drove straight to the main hospital unit, the Ife State hospital, where I informed my wife Dorothy of the situation before presenting myself before the two-member interim administration that had been overseeing the then hapless institution. Here was I, placed in supreme control of four hospitals and three health centres, with over 2,000 members of staff and over 500 beds. Prior to this, I had not even administered a department!

The two Ministry of Health officials handed over hurriedly and were gone the following day. The briefing was minimal and there were no hand-over notes. The Director of Clinical Services, who also had the title of Chairman, Medical Advisory Committee (CMAC), and who had been centrally involved in the dispute on the CMD's side, was clearly unenthusiastic about my appointment. The Assistant Director of Administration, Gbadebo Ibuoye, who had been appointed Acting Director by the Government, was more helpful, and provided a fuller picture of the state of affairs. The picture he painted was of demoralised staff, split down the middle into supporters of the hastily retired Director of Administration and those of the terminated CMD. Salaries had not been paid for two months and the institution was literally not functioning.

The priorities were clear: pay salaries, get the institution back on its feet and unite the sectionalised workforce. I stated these priorities in meetings with the various staff unions and during meetings with Heads of Departments within the institution. As stated earlier, my appointment had not been received with enthusiasm by the staff, and quite rightly so—I was not well-known and had no administrative experience. I did have one major advantage though—I had never been identified with either of the two factions. Indeed, both Dorothy, a radiologist, and I had distanced ourselves from the dispute, and had gone on working when almost everyone else in the hospital was on strike. Although the former CMD and his close associates looked at me with suspicion, most of the other workers were able to regard me as neutral in the conflict, and I believe the meetings I held with them went some way in convincing them that I was a fair-minded person with no other objectives than to re-motivate the staff and get the hospital back to work. The Ife University Teaching Hospitals Complex comprises several units, and to refer to it as a "hospital" would therefore be a misnomer. Nevertheless, for convenience, it shall be described as "the hospital" from here on—apologies to sticklers for semantics.

We were fortunate to have a committed and capable Chief Accountant in the person of Yemi Ogunjimi. We went through the accounts of the hospital together, and by scraping funds together from the various accounts, we were able to find enough money to make up the "take-home" pay of the staff. The outstanding salaries were paid immediately, but we could not pay out on tax, union dues and other deductions—debts that normally should only be accumulated as a last resort. However, this was certainly justified in this particular desperate situation. The effect of paid salaries on staff morale was predictable and full services were restored in the hospital within a very short time.

The ten-month period of the "Acting Administration" is merely the beginning of my story. Nevertheless even in that short space of time, there were some developments that must be mentioned.

Perhaps most important is that the period marked my baptism in administration. Having had no previous training in administration, I learnt the hard way, on the job, and from my successes as well as my mistakes. In particular, I learnt how to motivate people. In retrospect, it is difficult to say how I achieved this; I believe it came naturally. The important factors probably include a genuine commitment to the hospital and the welfare of its staff, and being able to convey this to them, so that they believed in me. Of course, no one is perfect, but I tried to be as fair to everyone as is humanly possible. I also hope that I was able to convey to them the true values that I hold dear—hard work, honesty and honour; values that, alas, are so rare in our country today. I believe this approach not only motivated the staff but also resolved the polarisation that had been so prominent during the crisis.

I was not a particularly good planner; I still am not, but, working with the staff, we were able to determine our priorities for the success of the institution. The things that make a good hospital are not an array of sophisticated and expensive equipment, but much more basic things like cleanliness, water and power supply, availability of drugs and other medical items, and prompt attention to patients, particularly in emergencies. Also, the need to ensure that patients, and their loved ones, feel that they are treated well. For all of these, you need a fulfilled and motivated workforce.

Initially, there was no Board of Management for the hospital, and along with the other teaching hospitals at that time, we were supervised by the Federal Ministry of Health. This necessitated frequent visits to the Ministry, then located in Ikoyi, Lagos. We received much support from the two Ministry officials who had served on the Interim Administration, Dr. Clement Orimolade and Mr. J.A. Akinyemi. They provided good advice, and also smoothed the path of bureaucracy, a phenomenon that I was not familiar with. A family friend, Mrs. Aisha Rahaman, who was an administrator in the hospital, was close to the seat of Government and was also very helpful in our dealings with the Ministry. Incidentally, Aisha was also one of my most trusted advisers throughout the period of my acting administration as well as one of the most indispensable administrators—a truly capable woman.

Water supply was a major problem in all the hospital's units. Much of the supply was by tanker. A young doctor introduced me to the Director of the Ogun–Osun River Basin Development Authority, which had been developing its borehole drilling services. I obtained quotations from them for feasibility studies and drilling of boreholes in each of the units and took them to the Ministry. Mr. Akinyemi rushed through the approval and the contracts were awarded. The first borehole was drilled in the Ife State Hospital unit and was extremely successful. That borehole is still functioning to this day. The other three boreholes were less successful; the one at the Wesley Guild Hospital was a total failure and two others provided minimal yield. However, it was a good start, and from that time, boreholes have been the main source of water supply to the institution. The exception is the Wesley Guild Hospital and this will be commented on more elaborately later. We overhauled all the generators and were able to greatly improve the power supply to all the units.

Throughout the period of my acting administration, the hospital was under-funded. The total annual budget for 1984 was ₦8.7 million, which was ₦1 million less than the wage bill. This dire situation extended to all the teaching hospitals, and in almost all of them, the staff were owed arrears of salaries. The Military Government addressed this problem with characteristic military fashion. They put some funds together and sent contingents of the army to pay the outstanding salaries in each hospital, based on a "show your face" staff audit. The exercise was to be coordinated by the military governors in each state. The exact amount owed each member of staff was paid, based on documented evidence of non-payment. This arrangement created a serious problem for us, since we had paid all the outstanding arrears of salaries by scraping together funds from the institution's various accounts. "Trouble *don* come!". I was now in despair for fear that we were going to lose money. To solve the problem, I drove down to Ibadan to see the Military

Governor, Colonel Oladayo Popoola. As I proceeded to explain my predicament, I was astounded at how quickly he grasped the seriousness of the situation. I have not met anyone before or since quicker to assess the gravity of a situation. Talk about the incisive military mind! We agreed on a solution, which was to provide documents on the payments we had made and which would then be reimbursed to the hospital. This is exactly what we did when the army officers arrived in the hospital three days later. I have held Colonel (now retired General) Popoola in very high regard since then. A few months later, both of us came near to being dismissed over our handling of a doctors' strike.

My first experience of the machinations of trade unions occurred soon after I got into office. For many years, the institution had four trade unions; actually two unions and two staff associations, since two of them were not registered. The junior staff and a few senior staff came under the Non-Academic Staff Union of Educational and Associated Institutions (NASU) and the nurses and midwives belonged to the National Association of Nigerian Nurses and Midwives (NANNM); both registered trade unions. There was also the Senior Staff Association of Teaching Hospitals, Universities and Research Institutes (SSATHURAI) and the Resident Doctors Association.

One morning, I received a letter from a new union called the Medical and Health Workers Union of Nigeria (MHWUN) stating that it now had jurisdiction over the junior staff and announcing that it intended to hold a congress in the institution. NASU had heard about this and was furious. Militant pronouncements were made and there were some clashes in the hospital between NASU hardliners and the self-appointed leaders of the fledgling MHWUN. As if we did not have enough troubles, the problem coincided with the arrival of the soldiers charged with the payment of our salary arrears. Some hospital workers, I presume members of the NASU executive, briefed the officer in charge of the army team of the situation and he promptly arrested the MHWUN leaders and took them to the police headquarters in Ile-Ife. That was the end of the problem! Human rights? Anyway, I wasn't complaining!

The financial situation in the institution was quite grim throughout the period of my acting administration. Salaries had to be scraped together at the end of each month, and there was virtually nothing left for anything else. We could hardly stock any drugs, and patients had to purchase most of their medicines and other requirements from nearby pharmacies, which did a roaring trade. We had a consultant obstetrician, Professor J.A. Akingba, who had retired from Ibadan and was on contract with us. One day while we were discussing the problem of our inability to stock drugs, he suggested that I should copy the system that had been operating in the Igboora Community Health Project many years ago, whereby patients paid for their drugs and the money realised was used to replenish stocks. A similar system had been established in the University of Benin Teaching Hospital for out-patients.

I immediately bought the idea. We had a military government, which was fond of drastic procedures for getting things done. One of its favourite strategies was to use "task forces." I liked the idea of task forces, because to my mind, they would be able to get things done without the encumbrance of bureaucratic procedures. I set up a task force, involving two pharmacists, an accountant and a surgeon, all of whom had demonstrated at one time or the other that they had the drive as well as the integrity to succeed. Within a month, the "Pharmacy Shop" was opened to much fanfare. It operated strictly on a cash-for-goods basis. The operational system is best defined in terms of the old adage "Money for hand, back for ground". It succeeded beyond our wildest dreams. High quality drugs and other essential medical items were available at very good prices. This was possible because all the overheads were paid by the hospital, including the salaries of the staff. Thus, the Drug Revolving Fund was born. This system has since been copied all over the country and beyond. The history of the Drug Revolving Fund and of the revolving funds for other medical items that were also introduced subsequently, began with this first small "Pharmacy Shop". Dedicated, honest people made it possible—Mrs. Gbonju

Ayoola, Mrs. Ilemabode Nwakpa, Mr. David Imafidon and Dr. Soji Oluwole.

I found the singular success of the Pharmacy Shop truly encouraging. I therefore took the opportunity of the commissioning ceremony of the Pharmacy Shop to set up four more task forces, charged with solving some major problems in the hospital. None of these task forces actually functioned. Indeed, the Chairman of one of them, an orthopaedic surgeon, did not even acknowledge the appointment, much less get going on the task. However, the announcement stung two senior officers into action. Both saw the establishment of the task force as reflecting negatively on their abilities, since the tasks were related to their own functions. They each promptly set about solving their two problems. One wrote to me within 48 hours stating that the problem had been resolved and that no task force was necessary! There are many ways to motivate people.

In the first quarter of 1985, the Nigerian Medical Association (NMA) embarked on a strike. The crisis started at the Lagos University Teaching Hospital over a relatively small matter that could easily have been resolved if it had been dealt with more appropriately at the outset. Resident doctors in that institution got angry over the sudden cancellation of one of their conditions of service. Their protests over this breach went unanswered and they got angrier. Over the course of the next week or so, they added to this grievance, complaints concerning lack of facilities in the teaching hospital. This was a time when all the hospitals were cash-strapped, and when, after salaries were just barely paid, virtually nothing was left to provide services to the patients. Operations and investigations were being severely curtailed and patients had to purchase almost everything required for their treatment from local shops. The staff were being paid, albeit often late, but did not have the tools they needed to perform their duties. Oddly, this was the situation in spite of the claim by the Head of State that a major reason for the military takeover was to reverse our hospitals being "virtually dispensing clinics!" Resident doctors in other teaching hospitals took up the cry, and the NMA waded into the case. The firebrand, Beko Ransome-

Kuti, was Chairman of the Lagos Branch of the NMA at that time; however, he emerged as the true leader of subsequent nationwide industrial action. The government was given an ultimatum to improve the services in the teaching hospitals or face total strike action. The soldiers did not respond and the NMA went on total strike, which shut down most government hospitals in the country.

The Government responded to the strike in typical military fashion. The NMA was proscribed and arrest orders were issued on its leaders as well as those of the Resident Doctors Association. A good number were arrested, and the others, including Beko, went into hiding. When I heard about the proscription over the radio, I went to look for the branch chairman of our residents. I found him packing out of his house, about to go into hiding. He expressed his determination and that of his colleagues to fight the government to the bitter end. That chairman was Bode Balogun, a brilliant young doctor, who subsequently became a Professor of Cardiology and later Provost of the College of Health Sciences. All but two of the junior doctors in the hospital stopped work. I met with the consultants, who agreed to man emergency services, and we kept the Accidents and Emergencies Units and Children's Emergency units open for a day or two, until they also joined the strike.

In response to the strike, the heads of all the teaching hospitals were called to an emergency meeting in Lagos. The Federal Minister of Health was Emmanuel Nsan, himself a doctor. Although he participated in the meeting, it was clear that he was not in charge. That "honour" belonged to a Colonel of the Engineering Corps, who declared in no uncertain terms that the doctors' strike would be quashed. He asserted that the strike was engineered by a group of socialist miscreants who were hell-bent on overthrowing the Government. I was the most junior head there as a result of the circumstances of my appointment. The rest were mainly provosts and deans, and thus professors. Nevertheless, I stood up and asserted that the striking doctors' only desire was for an improvement in the facilities in the hospitals, so that meaningful patient care could be provided. The military team sneered at my apparent naivety and I was surprised that even the civilian ministry officials seemed to agree with the soldiers' stance. None of my senior colleagues said a word. They all listened to the orders of the soldiers and left. The orders were to dismiss all the striking doctors and eject them from their quarters.

Two days afterwards, a friend came into my house in the university campus early in the night and told me that some policemen were outside in a Land Rover. I didn't believe I had done anything that warranted arrest or prosecution, so I waited. A police officer came in and informed me that the Military Governor had sent for me. The Land Rover team had been sent as a security escort. This was a time when it was not safe to drive on the highway at night because of armed robbers. This is still the case more than twenty-five years on. We left at about 9pm and arrived in the Governor's residence an hour later. I was immediately ushered into the presence of the Governor, who received me with the same courtesy that he had accorded me on our previous meeting. One thing I can say with certainty about military officers is that almost invariably they do live up to their reputation as "Officers and Gentlemen." He asked for a briefing on the situation in the hospital. He then gave instructions that any doctor who was on strike should be issued with a letter of dismissal and ejected from government quarters. He also requested for regular reports on the situation. I got back to Ife at around midnight.

The strike went on all over the country. I ordered the Acting Director of Administration to issue letters of dismissal to all the doctors who were on strike, but we could not deliver the letters since, as we claimed, they had left without any forwarding address. A few of the junior doctors, medical officers and resident doctors, put up irregular appearances at the hospital. The consultants held honorary appointments. Their full-time jobs were with the University. The consultants claimed they were working but in reality they were not, and, in any case, they could not realistically function without the residents. I wrote a report that all the consultants were at work and that a substantial number of the junior doctors had returned to work. The Governor received similar reports from the other teaching hospital in the State, the University College Hospital, Ibadan. He passed on the report that the two institutions were functioning to the Federal Government. Towards the end of the crisis, the Government sent a high ranking Air Force officer, a doctor, to confirm the position in Oyo and Kwara states. He visited the teaching hospitals in Ilorin and Ibadan and found that, contrary to the reports by the governors of the two states, the institutions were not functioning and that virtually every doctor was on strike, including the consultants. He did not visit Ile-Ife. I met this officer at a meeting in the Bonny Camp military cantonment in Lagos a couple of weeks later and he told me that the reason he did not visit Ile-Ife was that the Ife–Ibadan road was notorious for accidents. Besides which, he said that there had been so much trouble in Ife recently, referring to the prolonged crisis in the institution, saying that "your people must be tired of trouble". The two CMD/Deans in Ibadan and Ilorin, both colleagues of mine from the University of Ibadan, were dismissed. The Military Governor later told me that he had also been in hot water and was lucky to have extricated himself. But for the fear of our notorious road, I would presumably also have been dismissed.

One Sunday morning during the middle of the NMA strike, just when I was about to go fishing, the Acting DA arrived in my house in a state of extreme agitation. He said that the Director of Clinical Services, Professor Gani Ladipo, had been taken away by security men. Gani was the Deputy Chairman of the Nigerian Medical Association in Oyo State, and it was assumed that this was why he had been whisked away. I travelled down to Ibadan with Mr. Ibuoye to look for him. Our first stop was at the Governor's Lodge. We had obviously interrupted His Excellency's weekend recreation, but he received us. He was not sure exactly where Professor Ladipo was, but said it was likely he had been arrested as a security measure. The Police Headquarters would probably know his exact whereabouts. We drove to the Police HQ at Iyaganku, but the missing person was not there. A helpful officer suggested we try the NSO (National

Security Organisation) headquarters. We proceeded to the NSO state headquarters in Eleyele where we saw Gani's car parked. We were told that he was, indeed, in custody there. We found him in a sitting room, along with the State Chairman of the NMA, Dr. (Chief) Mrs. Tinuola Abiola-Oshodi and her husband, a retired police officer. Incidentally, that was my first meeting with Dr. Abiola-Oshodi, the woman who was to become a highly trusted friend and adviser and Chairman of the hospital's Management Board. We confirmed that both arrested persons were safe and in good health, and the officer-in-charge informed us that they had been arrested in order to break up communication within the leadership of the striking doctors.

We returned to Ile-Ife in better spirit. As soon as we got back, we went to Professor Ladipo's house to inform his wife that all was, at least relatively, well. Her response was to turn on me with great hostility, repeatedly shouting that "The truth will (be) out". I am still not sure why she thought I was involved in Gani's arrest; perhaps she thought I regarded him as a rival for the headship of the hospital. Her hostility still made no sense to me. We visited the two detainees in their confinement regularly until they were finally released a week later, by which time the strike had collapsed.

The Military Government had embarked on a war of attrition against the striking doctors. It ordered the arrest of the NMA and Resident Doctors' leaders, many of whom, including my colleague Gani Ladipo, were detained, but it had also ordered the ejection of the doctors from their quarters, and, more importantly, following their dismissal, had withheld their salaries. The strike collapsed after five weeks, and the Government ordered that they should only be reabsorbed after they had applied for re-employment and were formally interviewed. The Military Governor set up a team comprising a military officer, myself and some Oyo State Ministry of Health officials to interview all the dismissed doctors in the State, who were, in fact, the majority. Interviews were organised in the State Ministry of Health in Ibadan and in our headquarters unit in Ile-Ife. We conducted the interviews in batches. I have never participated in a strike action in my whole life; nevertheless, I found the humiliation that these doctors went through terrible. They included consultants in State Hospitals, some of whom were very senior to me. The consultants in my hospital were not affected, because the Government had not discovered that my claim that they had worked during the period of the strike was not true.

The NMA strike of 1985 was a different strike from all the others that have occurred in the country. It is the only strike action in the history of Nigeria that was not about pay rises. The doctors went on strike to improve the facilities in the hospitals. Beko Ransome-Kuti, who died in 2006, led that strike. The action was typical of him. He was prepared to sacrifice his freedom and even his life in the cause of social justice. He took this risk repeatedly throughout his life. May he rest in peace.

In the second quarter of 1985 following the strike, the Government issued Decree 10, which, as described earlier, is the most important law regulating the administration of teaching hospitals. The new full-time Chief Medical Directors provided for by the decree were not appointed immediately. However, new boards of management were appointed for each of the hospitals. The Chairman of the Board of Management of the Ife University Teaching Hospitals Complex was Colonel G.O. Emodi, an army doctor. When I look back on that board, the only member I remember clearly is Colonel Emodi. He was a colourful, forceful individual with clear ideas of how the institution should be run. The other members of the Board occupied the back stage. The Chairman quickly deployed to the hospital and worked closely with me. We agreed fully on what needed to be done to develop and sustain the institution. However, we lacked the funds to implement most of what we knew to be necessary. Indeed, one of his preoccupations was to retrench a substantial proportion of the workers, in line with the Government's belief that all the government-owned institutions were overstaffed. The Government had issued a directive to retrench a significant number of the non-professionals. We never did actually implement this directive before I was unceremoniously removed from office a couple of months later. That notwithstanding, while Colonel Emodi was the Chairman, there was discipline in the institution and the staff knew that the hospital was moving in a positive direction. I personally found him to be honest and committed to bringing value to the services of the Institution.

On the lighter side, Colonel Emodi very much enjoyed his Gulder beer. He had me in good company. Dorothy and I liked him a lot. My only regret was that I was not able to work with him for longer.

I have described some of the notable occurrences of the ten-month period. However, these events do not fully represent the achievements of the period. There was virtually no money, so physical development was at a standstill. What we were able to achieve was a substantial improvement in services, based on making what was available work well. Having put the polarity of the past behind them, the staff made a united effort to make everything in the hospital work. The hospital was clean, water and power supply were improved, and though this was not perfect, patients were treated promptly and, more importantly, in a humane manner. The pharmacy shop revolving fund system improved the supply of drugs and medical items. There was discipline, instilled not by threats of punishment but out of a genuine desire for efficiency. The staff knew that they were guaranteed fairness and justice when issues came up. From the security guards to the top health professionals, we were proud of the work we did and proud of the Ife University Teaching Hospitals Complex.

With the promulgation of Decree 10, I knew that a new Chief Medical Director would soon be appointed. I believed that I stood a good chance of being the one. When I received a letter from the Ministry enquiring as to whether I would be interested in the job, I showed it to the Acting DA. His advice was that I should first of all request for the conditions attached to the post. I foolishly took his advice and replied to this effect, rather than state that I was indeed interested. This gave the Ministry the excuse to say that I was not really interested in the job. I kept on working and working very hard, not knowing that various individuals were lobbying for the job. When the announcement was made on the appointment of the new CMD, I was the only one who was surprised. The adage about monkeys and baboons is possibly applicable! I did not understand the politics of such appointments, but then I have never engaged in politics over my personal fortunes. I never shall.

After what amounted to a dismissal over the radio, I went back to my home on the university campus. I informed Dorothy, who was furious at the manner of the announcement. I applied for a sabbatical and went off to Aberdeen for a year. I never received any acknowledgement from the Government for the service I had rendered in helping to get a crisis–ridden institution back to work. A few months after I was removed over the radio, the Management Board did write a letter of appreciation to me. I had developed a great love for the hospital and continued to believe that one day I would return as CMD. True indeed, I did return, four years later.

II

Acting Again

After my one-year sabbatical, I returned to my job as Consultant Psychiatrist in the Faculty of Health Sciences. I had now been promoted Professor, backdated to 1 October 1984. Both the University and the Hospital had been re-named in honour of Chief Obafemi Awolowo, who died in 1987. I also continued with my work as an honorary consultant in the hospital, in my beloved psychiatric unit at the Wesley Guild Hospital in Ilesa. At the end of 1988, I was appointed Acting Secretary-General of the West African College of Physicians, and subsequently Secretary-General, and this took up a substantial amount of my time. My hands were full.

Sometime in late August 1989, I was at a meeting of the West African Health Community when Dr. Tom Chiori, who was the chairman of the meeting in his capacity as Director of Medical Services of the Federal Ministry of Health, asked me, "Roger, have you received the letter?" I said that I had not received any letter, at least not from the Ministry. He told me that the letter was very important and that he would get his secretary to provide a copy. The copy came just as the meeting was ending. It read:

> *His Excellency, the President of the Federation, has approved your appointment as Acting Chief Medical Director of the Obafemi Awolowo University Teaching Hospitals Complex with immediate effect.*

Professor Gani Ladipo, the former Medical Director, had completed his term and left two months earlier, and there was much speculation over who would be appointed in his place. I knew that I was in the running, but naturally many others wanted the job too. There was a lot of lobbying in high places, and those who had religious connections were organising prayers and fasting. Although I wanted the job, I had not gone to see anyone to influence the decision or to seek divine intervention.

I got to know much later that some individuals from the hospital and from the Ile-Ife community, unknown to me, had approached the Minister of Health, Professor Olikoye Ransome-Kuti, and told him how well I had performed during my ten-month stint such that when he was presented with the names of all the shortlisted professors in the Faculty of Health Sciences, it was said that he pointed at my name and said, "This is the one I want." Thereafter, my name was presented to the Head of State for approval.

I went back to Ile-Ife with the copy of the letter, but by the next morning I found the original copy. Armed with this copy, I drove to the Hospital's headquarters. By the time I arrived, nobody else had heard about the appointment. The letter broke the news and I was received with much jubilation. While it was only an acting appointment until a substantive Chief Medical Director was appointed, it was clear that if I did well, I could get the full appointment.

With the goodwill of virtually all the members of staff, and my own enthusiasm, I set to work. I had no pre-designed plan. All I desired was to make the hospital work, and work better. I was basically concerned with what are considered to be the basic standards for a good hospital.

Motivating the members of staff was a major priority. For a number of years, promotions had been frozen as a result of the need to reduce costs. Quite a number of individuals therefore, had been stagnating in their posts for years. I therefore set out to put that right in the first exercise by recommending a large number of individuals to the Management Board and its Establishments' Committee for promotion. The worried Chairman asked me, "Can you afford the cost of all these promotions?" I answered that we could.

There is a widely held view, even in government circles, that promotions should be restricted because of their cost. In fact, on average, only a third of the salary increase on a promotion is the result of the promotion itself—the other two-thirds were from the annual increment, which the individuals would earn whether they were promoted or not. More importantly, in my view, the benefits to the institution from the motivational effects of the promotions far outweighed this "cost." The lesson here is that you promote only those who really deserve to be promoted as a result of their performance. If promotions are granted as a routine, e.g., because people have spent a specific number of years in their posts, then the value of the promotion as a motivational factor is lost. Anyway, we promoted a record number of staff, and the effect on morale and productivity in the hospital was considerable.

The Chairman of the Management Board was Professor (Chief) J.O. Falaye, a retired gastroenterologist. He had spent a short period as Chairman of the Governing Council of the University and had been removed. How he got to be appointed Chairman of our Board soon afterwards came as a surprise to me. At each meeting of the Board, he would travel down with a retinue of hangers-on, and they partied every night in the Chairman's Lodge into the wee hours of the night. In fact, some members of staff organised parties for them. We did not get on well, but maintained a polite tolerance for each other.

A member of the Board who was markedly different was Dr. (Chief) Mrs. Tinu Abiola-Oshodi, the representative of the Nigerian Medical Association (NMA). She was Chairman of the Establishments Committee, and showed a total dedication to fairness and justice in her dealings. On the main Board, she demonstrated an extraordinary understanding of the requirements for the delivery of good medical care. She was an obstetrician who had worked for many years with the Western Region Government and, subsequently, the Oyo State Government and so had acquired a wealth of experience in hospital administration. She came on board as a professional with a vast experience. She also came across as being absolutely honest.

When the time for the appointment of a new Board of Management for the Teaching Hospitals was approaching, there was much speculation as to who the new people would be. I assumed that a new Chairman would be appointed for the hospital, and my overriding desire was that Dr. Abiola-Oshodi should remain on the Board. The decision on who should represent the NMA on the management board was entirely theirs. Nevertheless, I mentioned the matter to the Minister, Professor Olikoye Ransome-Kuti, during an audience with him. He promised to have a word with the NMA. During the next meeting of the Board, Professor Falaye spoke in a manner that made it clear to everyone that he was going to be re-appointed. I spoke to the Ministry's representative on the Board, Dr. Ajayi-Obe, who confirmed that Professor Falaye's name was indeed on the list of the proposed board chairmen that was going to the Head of State for approval. I was filled with concern because we did not share common values and views on how the hospital should be managed. I decided to take action.

I travelled to Lagos to see the Minister, Olikoye Ransome-Kuti in his office at about 7am. This was the best time to see him, provided he let you in. He allowed me. I pleaded for forgiveness for disturbing him so early. Actually, I made the same 7am expedition many times afterwards but he always let me in. "Sir," I told him, "I had some information that Professor Falaye may be re-appointed as Chairman of our Board. I just want to let you know that I have some serious concern as we do not share the same objectives with respect to patient care and hospital management." The Minister thanked me for the insight but did not say a word about his intention. I left satisfied that I had at least done what I should. Members of the new board were announced ten days later. Dr. Abiola-Oshodi was our new Chairman! I instantly knew we had a frame for a good Board.

At the time of her appointment, Dr Abiola Oshodi was in her early sixties. She was totally committed to the good of the institution. She had retired from Government service a few years earlier with a reputation as one of the finest doctors in Oyo State. She had been responsible for the safe delivery of a good number of the babies in Ibadan, and after she retired from government service, she had a successful private medical practice that was widely known. As a result of this, she was warmly received in just about every home in Ibadan, a fact that we exploited to the full when we launched our development fund later. She faced her task with absolute commitment. She knew what was required of a good health institution and pursued this with single-mindedness throughout her tenure as Chairman. She not only shared my values—hard work, honesty, honour—she epitomized them. I will illustrate this with just one case: when we were working to get the Wesley Guild Hospital water scheme going, we were faced with an increase in the contract sum that had been awarded by the Board because of a sharp increase in the price of steel reinforcement. The added cost of this material, which constituted a major component of the project, was going to raise the contract sum by over one million naira. The Chairman travelled with me for three whole days in order to obtain the support of all the Board members for the new contract sum. She tirelessly undertook the assignment with me.

She paid particular attention to what was going on in the wards, with frequent unscheduled visits during which she would interact with both staff and patients. She could not stand even a hint of corruption. On one occasion she personally reprimanded a Board member who had gone to one of our service companies and organised a job for his own company. In her earlier career, she had been nicknamed *Ese ya ju moto* (Her feet are faster than a motor car) at the Adeoyo State Hospital, Ibadan. I soon found out why. When she moved around the hospital, it was at a truly hectic pace. Even I, much taller, had difficulty keeping up with her pace. She was honest to a fault, and had impeccable morals.

The events in the Chairman's Lodge that were associated with her predecessor's tenure were replaced by quiet nights with her grandson, whom she would bring with her to each board meeting.

Then there was Chief (Dr.) J.O. Toyosi, the new NMA representative. My first impression of him was of a noisy, bombastic gentleman, and I was rather pessimistic about his potential. It turned out I was wrong. He was second only to the Chairman in his dedication and, with his practical knowledge of health care and its management, he proved an invaluable ally to the Chairman. He was a man of the highest integrity. His political acumen was invaluable when it came to dealing with staff matters, which proved extremely important in his function as the Chairman of the Establishments (Personnel Matters) Committee. I found him to be a truly likeable man. Whenever I went to Ibadan, I would stop at his house, and, having avoided assault by his ferocious German Shepherd, I would be served a slice of his wife's delicious home-made cake. Sadly, Mrs. Ingrid Toyosi died in 2005. She was such a delightful woman with a big heart. Chief Toyosi himself remained a friend to the day of his death from a protracted illness in 2009.

Mr. C.O. Oyediran, representing community interests, was a partner in one of the foremost accounting firms in the country. A quiet, decent individual, he made astute contributions to the Board's deliberations, and was extremely supportive of the Chairman and myself. There was also Prince Adeyera Adeyemo, an Ife indigene and prominent businessman. He provided major advice on financial matters, and in the execution of company deals. We actually did use the services of the companies recommended by him, believing he was trying to help. Quite understandably, he was particularly interested in furthering the fortunes of Ile-Ife and its indigenes.

Mallam Rana K. Mallum was from Jos. He was a very pleasant individual, but seemed to be somewhat reserved and reticent, almost at sea in some of our deliberations. In conversation with the Minister, I learnt that he had performed superbly as the principal of a School of Health Technology. The Board appointment was a reward for this. Apart from these individuals, we also had representatives of the Honourable Minister of Health, the State Ministry of Health, and the Association of Medical Laboratory Technologists. The Dean of the Faculty of Health Sciences (subsequently the Provost of the College), the VC's representative and the Chairman Medical Advisory Committee (CMAC) were also members of the Board. The Secretary to the Board was the Director of Administration (DA), a very pleasant and hard working individual named Lawrence Adeyeye. He had been appointed DA a few months before I arrived. He was a very pleasant man, easy to get on with, and quite humble. He did his job, and did it well. He was extremely loyal, both to the hospital and to me. All the internal members made very valuable contributions: Professor Kayode Adetugbo, Provost of the College of Health Sciences, was particularly effective, and also very supportive. Not surprisingly, we shared similar views and values.

The central administration of the hospital involved a three-man team—the CMD, the Chairman (CMAC) and the Director of Administration (DA).

The tenure of a CMAC is two years. It is renewable once, and I worked with a total of five of them. Dr. E.A. Bamgboye was the incumbent Chairman when I arrived, but his tenure ended within a few weeks. I then had to make a recommendation to the Board for a new Chairman. Dr. Layi Ige, a neurosurgeon, better known as "IG," had popular support within the hospital. I had known him for many years as a highly committed doctor of the highest integrity. We were both members of the OAU Staff Club. I took his name to the Board and he was appointed on 22 November 1989. We worked very well together. He knew what the priorities were, and shared my commitment to ensuring that the institution provided services of the highest quality. I was really happy with him.

On the morning of 29 September 1990, I made a quick trip to the Wesley Guild Hospital Unit. On my return at about 9.30 am, my secretary came running, saying IG was seriously ill. He had complained of feeling faint earlier that morning, and

Dr. Ade Ajayi, a cardiologist, had seen him in his home and advised that he be taken to hospital. As he was about to enter the ambulance, he collapsed. He was taken straight to the Accidents and Emergencies Department where a whole squad of doctors struggled to resuscitate him. His heart beat came back briefly, but his breathing never did. An electrocardiogram showed that he had suffered a massive myocardial infarction (heart attack). After two hours of resuscitation, he was pronounced dead. At his funeral in Edun Abon, a self-opinionated preacher made two unfortunate statements. During a tirade about poor facilities in the hospital he stated, "There are no drugs in that hospital." And this was when our innovative drug revolving fund was working so well and being copied by other hospitals. He then made matters worse when he stated that Layi never went to church. The Chaplain of the Church had to intercede and state that Layi had actually hosted the Church's Men's Fellowship the weekend before his death. I have never had any regard for that bigoted priest afterwards. Contrast this with Layi's Memorial Service a year later where the preacher, Reverend Ilutanmi, gave a brief but extremely impressive sermon in which he reflected accurately on Layi's qualities. Rev. Ilutanmi closed the sermon with an unforgettable question: "What will they say about you when you are gone?" I will always remember those words.

Dr. Dele Hamed was the Deputy Chairman and was appointed in IG's place. We worked well together, but not in the same way as I had done earlier with my friend. Dr. Hamed got a job in Saudi Arabia and left the institution on sabbatical leave. Dr. A.O. Oyelese followed; he also was committed and loyal, but without the fire of Layi. Finally there was David Akinola, a surgeon. He was once a deputy to Dr. Hamed. I knew him fairly well. We had worked together in the Wesley Guild Hospital. I had earlier appointed him Physician-in-Charge of that unit and he carried out the task commendably. I remember asking a close friend about him. That was Olu *(Oga)* Arigbabu, of whom more will be said later in this book. *Oga's* reply was, "Take him; you will never regret it". I never did regret it, he turned out to be a wonderful colleague-in-arms. He was full of enthusiasm and extremely capable; we got on very well together. I was delighted when he was appointed Chief Medical Director after me.

Aside from the two members of the top trio in the central management, I also had to work closely with a number of others. The Hospital, as I call it, is a multi-unit establishment, with two specialist divisions: the Wesley Guild Hospital in Ilesa and the Ife State Hospital in Ile-Ife, a dental hospital on the University campus, and health centres in Ile-Ife, Ilesa, and Imesi-Ile. In each we had a Management Team of Physician-in-Charge, Unit Matron, and Unit Administrator. We held meetings with each team once a month and these included a tour of the facilities. These meetings allowed the Central Administration to keep abreast of the situation in each unit and to resolve any problems that required our input. I remember, in particular, Dr. Soji Oluwole, who was for many years the Physician-in-Charge of the Ife State Hospital. Indeed, after Soji left, I took over as Physician-in-Charge myself, on his advice. David Akinola, Physician-in-Charge of the Wesley Guild unit, has already been mentioned.

Dr. A.O. Olusile was Physician-in-Charge of the Dental Hospital for most of the time that I was CMD. He was absolutely marvellous—dedicated, hard working, very capable, and with great human qualities. His commitment to the service of the Dental Hospital and the Faculty of Dentistry was at the cost of his own personal development. So committed was he that he did not make time to produce the academic publications that are required to achieve the rank of Professor. He was finally promoted Professor in 2006. When the promotion was announced, we were all truly delighted. The celebrations went on well into the night. Layi Olaniyi was Unit Administrator of the Ife State hospital for a period. He was the one with whom I worked to get the water problems sorted out in that unit. He was also instrumental to a number of other initiatives. The Oninure Fund, established to raise funds for needy patients, was his idea and he was instrumental to its success. Layi was sincerely truly committed, capable, and a truly good person. He subsequently rose to the position of Deputy Director of Administration—he thoroughly deserves it.

Mrs. Dorothy Ogedengbe was the Chief Matron of the Hospital until March 1993. She was replaced by Mrs. Josephine Adegbile. Both of them were fine examples of the true nursing tradition. Their duties as nurses were placed above everything else— the care of all the patients in the hospital was their only priority. They were not involved in unionism and strike actions, and shunned the perks of office that have become the priorities of senior nurses today. Their public and their personal lives were a reflection of true goodness. They fully deserved the fond appellation of "Mama." They were true Christians, not just because of their faith but also because of the exemplary lives they lived.

The hospital was fortunate to have a truly committed workforce. While they would not hesitate to protest in the most vigorous terms if they saw their rights being challenged, they were truly committed to the hospital, and, in particular, to the care of patients. One of the issues that I emphasised repeatedly was the role of all the staff in the provision of patient care. The message that I tried, and, I hope, succeeded in getting across was that every individual played an indispensible role in patient care, from the sanitary attendant to the most senior consultant. We paid particular attention to the welfare of the staff, and they all knew it. After one of our doctors nearly died from Hepatitis B infection, I went to the Board and convinced them of the need to immunise all our staff against this virus. It cost about US$75,000 at that time. Ours was the first ever health institution in the country to immunise all our staff against Hepatitis B. Finally, the members of staff saw clearly that we were committed, transparent and giving our best.

Of course, there were individuals who, one way or another, did not come on board with me. One was an administrator, and a senior one at that. My first brush with him was when he tried, surreptiously, to instigate members of senior staff to embark on industrial action over a pay claim. A few months later, he persuaded the Senior Staff Association to report me to the Governor of Osun State for victimising him, and I was summoned to the State Security Service headquarters in Osogbo on that account. More details about this will be provided later.

A more serious affair was a protracted period of fraud by one of our senior officers and some of his henchmen. They had devised a means of inflating contracts and getting the contracts awarded to unscrupulous contractors, with whom they would share the loot. With the aid of the Quantity Surveyor, they would inflate the quantities on a project. When the Bill of Quantities went out to contractors, the favoured contractor, knowing that the quantities were inflated, would be able to put in a much lower bid than the others, knowing that, although he had submitted lower and unrealistic rates, he would make up for that through the inflated quantities. The guidelines for contract awards included a provision that bids must be within 10% of the Engineering Department's estimates. But with insider knowledge, the contractor would be able to make a submission as close to 10% as possible. With each certified payment, the staff involved would get their cut. The matter came to my knowledge when I called in a contractor who was behind schedule on his job. He complained of financial difficulties. When I pointed out that he was being paid promptly on certificates that were issued to him, he then disclosed that the senior officer had been making excessive demands for kickbacks which the contractor could not meet. He then revealed the whole story to me. I kept the matter to myself while I personally made some checks on the quantities on a number of contracts. I did this by measuring floor areas for terrazzo work; a relatively simple matter. I found overestimates on contracts and on valuation certificates of between 25% and 40%. I reported the matter to the Board of Management, which ordered an investigation. During the course of the investigation the three culprits, including the senior officer, disappeared. In the case of the senior officer, his was a real tragedy because I found him to be extremely competent professionally. He was the source of his own ruin, and of the others he had persuaded to join him in the scam.

On another occasion, a senior member of the Civil and Maintenance Department conspired with some others to break into the Tenders Box. After examining all the submitted tenders for a construction project, they amended the tender of a contractor with whom they had conspired so that that contractor's tender would be the lowest within the standard margin of 10% of the department's estimate.

There was also the case of a Senior Laboratory officer who allegedly printed his own receipts! He would issue his receipts to patients, carry out the electroencephalogram test, and pocket the money. We discovered the scam after we received a complaint that a junior officer in the department had demanded money from a patient. When confronted, the junior stated that his boss was much more guilty and was issuing his own receipts, whereas he had merely been demanding bribes! We got some of the receipts from patients' files, and confirmed that they were forged. The signatures on the receipts were clearly those of the Laboratory officer's. Being a criminal case, it was reported to the Police. The officer was immediately suspended. He was arrested, but to our surprise, he was not charged. The Police informed us that a handwriting expert had determined that the signatures on the receipts were not those of the officer! He retired with full benefits.

It must be emphasized that the vast majority of our staff were decent, honest individuals, who were truly committed to the institution. These cases of fraud and other forms of evil were the exception, rather than the rule.

III

Day-to-Day Hospital Management

❑ ❑ ❑ ❑ ❑ ❑ ❑ ❑ ❑ ❑ ❑

Earlier, I mentioned the important factors that make up a good hospital. Hospitals are not just about equipment and technology. Those are important, but are of little relevance if some basic and, in my view, essential facilities and services are not provided first. Indeed, the majority of cases in medicine can be diagnosed and treated using the most basic tools of the doctor—our hands, our eyes, our ears, and our noses, backed up by the thermometer, stethoscope, sphygmomanometer, and a diagnostic set. In the past, doctors also used their tongues, but we no longer do so, except perhaps on ourselves, in the privacy of our homes! One advantage that the Nigerian-trained doctors have is that, deprived of modern technology, they have to make use of their basic clinical skills, and are thus better–trained in these skills. Sadly today, many hospitals lack even some of these basic equipment. To crown it all, it is not uncommon for some hospital administrators to lay emphasis on computerized tomography machines and other sophisticated and highly expensive equipment. The health care system, like so many other sectors in Nigeria, is a perfect example of misplaced priorities.

Other facilities that make a good hospital include electricity and water supply, along with clean, pleasant surroundings. Functional toilets and bathing facilities are not just necessary in the interests of hygiene and sanitation, they are also highly valued by our patients. Then there are the human issues— patients should be treated with consideration and courtesy and health professionals should show compassion and empathy towards them. That "Ca (cancer) stomach in Bed 6" is actually "Mrs. Thomas, a human being in pain and distress, with a worried and distressed husband and children." Showing that you care (compassion) and that you understand what they are experiencing (empathy) are important attributes of a good health professional and a good health institution. A few minutes of sympathetic explanation to Mrs. Thomas and her relatives can make all the difference to them.

Our ability to provide efficient and effective patient care rests on ensuring that the materials required for effective clinical work are available—the drugs and other essential consumable items. Laboratory technologists and their equipment are useless unless the required chemicals are provided, and surgeons are equally ineffective if they do not have gauze and sutures. Finally, patients need to be attended to promptly, and particularly in emergencies, where they must be provided with care quickly and unconditionally.

Dr. Abiola-Oshodi's Management Board saw these issues as the priorities, and so did the entire workforce. We proceeded to pursue these objectives with utmost determination.

In 1989, there was no public water supply to any of the units. The main hospital, Ife State Hospital (ISH) had one borehole, the one drilled while I was temporarily in charge in 1984, serving mainly the "Phase II" building. The rest of the hospital was supplied by water tanker. The other hospital unit, Wesley Guild Hospital, fared even worse. All supply was by tanker, often from Ife; the boreholes had not been successful. Boreholes had also been unsuccessful in the Eleyele Comprehensive Health Centre Unit. The only unit that had a reasonably good water supply was the Imesi-Ile Rural Comprehensive Centre. We contracted for a further three boreholes in the Ife State Hospital Unit, and one each in the Multipurpose Unit in Ilesa and the Comprehensive Health Centre in Ife. These boreholes provided all the water we needed in those units. Our engineering staff then installed networks of pipelines and surface tanks from which the water was pumped into the wards. A 24-hour supply was achieved in those units.

Wesley Guild Hospital was a more difficult problem. Apart from the two failed boreholes, one of which was donated by Dr. Lawrence Omole, we also resuscitated a series of deep wells, but to no avail. Dr. Lawrence Omole was one of the greatest benefactors of the hospital, and also a source of great encouragement and support to me personally; a truly great man. When the Methodist Mission owned and managed the hospital, they had also tried unsuccessfully to resolve the water problem. We had almost resigned ourselves to ever getting water supply to the hospital, until I had a chance meeting in the Chief Engineer's office with Engineer O.B. Adeyemi, the owner of a firm of water engineering consultants that had previously done some work for the institution. I mentioned the problem to him, and he asked, "Why don't you dam the Omi Ayao stream?" This stream passed through the hospital grounds. I laughed. To me, the stream was so tiny and I didn't see it supplying water to a bungalow, much less a hospital. However, he assured me that it could supply enough. There and then, we agreed that his firm should carry out a survey and produce a proposal.

Shortly afterwards, I received the proposal. A weir would be constructed on the stream, from which water would be pumped into an impoundment and then processed. A mini-treatment plant would be constructed, employing slow sand filtration, which was much cheaper than the conventional rapid filtration process. The cost was to be half a million naira. I took the proposal to the Minister. He promptly agreed to provide a special grant for the project, saying, "Roger, by the time this goes to contract, prices will have gone up; you will need three-quarters of a million." A month later, we received the cheque in full. There was a small hiccup. The dry season had arrived and we noticed that the water flow in the stream was much reduced. I measured the flow—a simple process—you time the passage of a float along a measured length of the stream and also measure the cross-sectional area of the stream. I confirmed that the flow was inadequate. The consultant modified the plan to replace the weir with a dam. The reservoir thus created would remove the necessity for a separate sedimentation impoundment. By the time the plans were ready, the cost of building materials and labour had risen. I returned to the Minister, who agreed to provide the further three-quarters of a million naira required. Once more, the cheque arrived promptly. The matter was now in the hands of the Management Board. They adopted the proposal enthusiastically, and we advertised for tenders. We received three quotations, ranging from ₦3.5 million to ₦7 million. The lowest was by a firm called La Mod Engineering Services, owned by Engineer Bashiru Mohammed. We negotiated with him and agreed on a final figure of ₦3 million. This man is one in a million, a true professional and an impeccably honest individual. The final price did go up, because of further rises in the price of steel reinforcement and cement, and we ended up with a cost of just over four million naira. The water works were finally commissioned in July 1992, and it provided all the water the hospital needed. Once the pipelines and surface tanks had been rehabilitated and upgraded, water flowed in all the wards.

Electricity was less of a problem. We were fortunate that a number of high-capacity generators had been procured in the 1980s. All that was required was to overhaul and maintain them. The cost of diesel had risen progressively over the years, and there had been frequent national shortages, but we managed to ensure supply most of the time. We sometimes had difficulty in keeping the units in Ilesa and Imesi-Ile supplied with diesel, since the fuel had to be taken to those units from Ife in a tractor tanker. One night in September 1993, I received a phone call from a senior resident doctor that there was no diesel for the generator in Wesley Guild Hospital, and some women in labour needed emergency operations. The junior staff were on strike at the time, and I initially said there was nothing that could be done, but, after some thought, I decided to take a drum of diesel there myself. I phoned the doctor and informed him of the plan. I drove to the Ife State Hospital, loaded the "Baby - Friendly" Land Cruiser with the diesel, and drove to Ilesa. To my disappointment, by the time I arrived, the consultant on duty had discharged the patients. What a contrast between this impatient consultant whose reaction was to send the patients away and the resident who took it upon himself to try to solve the problem by contacting me. I was never able to take that consultant seriously after that incident. The resident concerned has since demonstrated his commitment to patient care repeatedly, and is now one of our most valued consultants.

How do you keep a hospital clean? It's not about equipment and materials. It is more about the commitment of people. Not just the cleaners and orderlies, but all the members of staff. When patients and their relatives see how committed the staff are to a clean environment, they also tend to play their part. Of course you do need some equipment and materials, and we made sure these were available. Indeed, we were criticised by many for spending a quarter of a million on wheeled dustbins. We used to organise a monthly environmental sanitation exercise in which all the staff participated in cleaning and tidying the wards, clinics, and offices as well as the surroundings. The exception was the doctors, most of whom appeared to see cleaning as being beneath them. These exercises had a direct impact; they also served to emphasise the importance of cleanliness and good sanitation. The morale of the cleaning staff was greatly boosted — we were showing them how important their job was, and that their tasks were not menial, but work in which everyone participated. The "Ward of the Month" trophy was introduced — the trophy was awarded on the basis not only of cleanliness but also on general atmosphere and achievements. It attracted fierce competition. Every Saturday morning, I would go round the main hospital in Ile-Ife examining how clean each ward was and commenting on my findings, giving small rewards to the orderlies and nurses whose wards were in particularly good condition. I paid particular attention to the toilets, and, in the case of the medical wards, to their isolation units. These are the areas that are most likely to be neglected. My evaluations were sometimes rather unfair, since I would look for dirt and dust in the highest places that the average person had difficulty in reaching! I am much taller than most people. On some weekends, I also went round the Wesley Guild Hospital and the comprehensive health centres. The units largely consisted of old buildings, but we kept them clean and attractive and the staff were very proud of this.

***   ***   ***

It has been mentioned that the hospital pioneered the establishment of a drug revolving fund. In subsequent years, the Federal Government actually adopted drug revolving fund schemes in all its health facilities. The official origin of this lies in the Bamako Agreement for providing drugs at the primary health care level, which, under Professor Ransome-Kuti's tenure, was expanded to include the Federal teaching and specialist hospitals through a scheme financed by the World Bank. We are not officially recognised as the source of this innovation; nevertheless, we do believe that our pioneering success was instrumental in influencing the development of the scheme— as it is often said, if you don't blow your own trumpet, who will blow it for you? We took the scheme much further, and decided to introduce revolving fund schemes for all systems that were dependent on consumable items such as dental materials, operating theatre materials (the "emergency pack" scheme), laboratory consumables, radiology ("X-Ray") materials, and medical consumables.

These schemes had a tremendous impact on the institution's services. Things got done, and emergencies were treated promptly and efficiently. We were proud of our record with emergencies, and even those who did not have the means to pay for emergencies were all treated without hesitation. It must be emphasised here that, even when we provided immediate care to emergency cases without pre-payment, the majority subsequently paid up. We received delegations from many other teaching hospitals who wanted to learn about our revolving fund schemes and who subsequently set up their own. There are some basic management principles that must be followed in order to ensure the success of a revolving fund. We shared our managerial expertise with them. Equally important is that the scheme must be run by committed and honest individuals.

Of course, facilities alone are not a guarantee of service delivery. The staff are critical to that, and so also is the manner in which the facilities are employed. I have already mentioned the importance we gave to motivating the staff. They knew that clinical services were our priority, and we emphasised this continually and also demonstrated it. I spent more time going round the wards, clinics, and service departments than I spent in the CMD's Office or the Board Room. My first port of call in the morning before I went to my office, was the Accidents' and Emergencies Department. Some days, I would drive to the hospital in the early hours of the morning and go round the hospital.

The hospital's fees were modest, but even then quite a few patients could not afford them. It was the practice in many hospitals to turn away patients who could not pay in advance for their treatment; even life threatening emergencies would be turned away. This was the case in the hospital when I took over. I put in place a regulation that all emergency cases should be treated, even when patients could not pay the fees. This regulation was generally adhered to. I say "generally," because of an incident that occurred in 1991. A member of the public wrote to the Ministry of Health complaining of gross neglect in the treatment of his sister who had died in the hospital. I investigated, and found that the lady, who had developed peritonitis as a result of typhoid fever, had spent several hours in the Accidents and Emergencies Department of the Ife Unit waiting for surgery. Her relatives had not paid for the materials required for the surgery. The staff of the Department had not released the materials because they believed the family was well-off and could pay. The delay in carrying out the operation certainly contributed to the death of the patient. One of the outcomes of this incident was that I further strengthened the regulation to the effect that, in emergency cases, treatment should be implemented immediately. The patient and carers should be informed of the cost, but treatment should go ahead without delay. Those who did not have the funds on them invariably paid later, and I believe the provision greatly contributed to the reputation of the institution.

We guaranteed immediate treatment for all emergency cases, however, that still left the care of less urgent cases. In any community, there is a proportion of genuinely poor individuals who cannot pay for their treatment. On an ad hoc basis, we would assess such individuals and provide for them if we confirmed that they genuinely could not pay. We also set up the *Oninure* (welfare) Fund to provide for the other needs of such patients. In this regard, as mentioned earlier, Mr. Layi Olaniyi, then a relatively young and junior administrator, played a key role.

Around 1990, a maternal death occurred in the Lagos University Teaching Hospital. Following a complaint by the patient's relatives of neglect by the obstetric team that had managed the case, an enquiry was set up. The enquiry found that there had been gross neglect in the management of the case and that the woman would not have died if prompt and appropriate treatment had been provided. Olikoye Ransome-Kuti, Federal Minister of Health, decided that from thereon all cases of maternal deaths should be reported to his Ministry. At that time, Dr. (now Professor) Friday Okonofua was the Head of the Obstetrics and Gynaecology Department. We set up a system of regular reviews of all maternal deaths. I attended majority of the reviews. I believe the move resulted in an improvement of our obstetric services, because the members of the department, both doctors and nurses, were aware of the interest of both the Ministry and the Hospital Administration in their performance. With only one exception, we were able to show that the management of these cases in the hospital was prompt and correct. The on-call system for the labour wards and maternity wards was effective; indeed, the resident doctors slept in on-call rooms within the labour wards. The Emergency Pack Revolving Fund system ensured the ready availability of the materials and drugs required for emergency operations. The major causes of maternal deaths were inadequate ante-natal care prior to arrival in the hospital and delay in the referral of the cases to us when complications had set in. Incidentally, referrals from health and maternity centres were sent direct to the labour wards and not through the Accident and Emergency departments. Only in one instance were we at fault in a case of maternal death. This was where both ureters (the tubes draining the kidneys) had been tied during the operation. We set up an official enquiry chaired by a very senior gynaecologist, Dr. R.A. Onifade. The enquiry found the consultant involved culpable. After the baby had been delivered, he had left a relatively junior resident doctor to complete the operation. The consultant was officially reprimanded by a panel of senior consultants.

IV

Managing Industrial Crises

One of the major themes that run through this book is the difficulties with the unions. With hindsight, I accept that many of these cases could have been handled better by me. I did not have too many local problems in the hospital, but there were a number of industrial actions at the national level. Over the years, I developed a very good relationship with most of the staff of the institution. There were obviously one or two exceptions—there always are; you can't please everybody all of the time. We gave priority to staff welfare, and they knew it, through promotions and other rewards, loan schemes, housing, etc., and also, by providing them with a conducive working environment and the requirements to do their work. Perhaps just as important, they came to believe that the administration I led, and the Abiola-Oshodi Management Board, were committed to ensuring that the services of the institution were of the highest standard and that we were not there to enrich ourselves. I believe the unions also believed in us and, for most of the time, they worked closely with the Administration and the Board, except, of course, when this did not suit their ends.

A few members of staff with grievances also tried, sometimes successfully, to use their union in the pursuit of their cause. The most obvious example of this was when I verbally reprimanded a Deputy Secretary for incompetence. He had gone to the Senior Staff Association and complained of victimisation. The Association had taken up the case by reporting me to the State Military Governor, who referred the case to the State Security Service. The first I knew about this was when an SSS officer came to my office and informed me that the State Director of the organisation was inviting me to his office in connection with the case. I told the officer that I was not coming. He expressed surprise and said he would return. I spoke to one of my closest friends, Professor ("Uncle") David Ijalaye, who advised me that I had better go or I might be taken there by force. I travelled to Osogbo and reported in the office of the Director at the State Headquarters. I explained the situation, I believe, to the Director's satisfaction; at least that is what he said. The Association's case was further worsened by the fact that it was not a registered trade union. It must be said that the Director treated me with the greatest courtesy. It was later discovered that the Deputy Secretary was secretly instigating the unions against the Administration in connection with their conditions of service—not what you would expect of a senior administrator. When, during the subsequent annual promotion exercise, I confronted him with this, he vigorously denied it, "As a member of the Administration, I could never do that." However, the external assessor, a senior administrator from the UCH, Ibadan, confirmed this and reminded him that he threw the Deputy Secretary out of his hospital when he came to mobilise the staff there on the same issue! He did not get promoted that year. He did eventually get promoted, and, long after I had left, ended up as Director of Administration, but later than he had planned!

The doctors went on strike three times during the eight-year period that I served as Chief Medical Director. Each one was horrific in its consequences. Ordered off by the National Association of Resident Doctors, or its parent body, the NMA, they would abandon work, leaving the sick on their hospital beds and the emergency services unattended. Sometimes the consultants provided skeletal services, but there was untold suffering, and each time, many patients would die. One story sticks in my mind. Just before the onset of a strike by the doctors sometime in 1995, a lady from Aba, eastern Nigeria arrived with her only son. She had been told that we were the only institution that could save her son's life. At that time we were the only public hospital with a dialysis unit and had already developed a reputation for our renal care services. He was admitted to the male medical ward. Before any treatment could commence, the doctors went on strike. Her grief was indescribable. I remember personally resuscitating him once when he went into a hypoglycaemic (low blood sugar) coma, assisted by a House Officer. The next day the young man again went into a coma, this time from renal failure, and died in spite of our efforts. He needed dialysis but this could not be done without the striking members of the renal team. Will that mother ever forgive us? On another occasion, during a strike by NASU, one of our most dedicated nurses died because we could not generate electricity to the operating theatre during a power failure. So much death resulting from humankind's inhumanity to humankind.

These deaths and the suffering by patients and their relatives are repeated all over the country's hospitals when doctors go on strike. And yet we swear to an oath when we qualify, which includes the statements, "The health of my patient shall be my first consideration" and "I will maintain the utmost respect for human life." Doctors justify strike action by contending that that is the only way to get through to the Government and that it is their right to go on strike. However, we all swore the Hippocratic Oath. When lecturers go on strike, students don't get taught and classroom losses can be made up for. When doctors go on strike, people die and there is untold suffering because death is irreversible.

The nurses were no better. When given the order by their very militant union, the National Association of Nigerian Nurses and Midwives (NANNM), they would all troop off, abandoning their patients, even in the middle of dressing their injuries. They would lock up everything and take away all the keys, including the keys to the drug cupboards and trolleys. When they went on strike, the concept of senior management being exempt from strikes was thrown by the wayside; you were lucky to have even the Director of Nursing Services staying at work. Those senior nurses who wanted to stay on and help patients were threatened with physical violence or *juju*. It is amazing how many Nigerians, even those highly educated, believe in the power of *juju*.The local situation was compounded by the fact that, the nurses also belonged to the Senior Staff Association of Universities, Teaching Hospitals and Research Institutes (SSAUTHRAI), so that even if NANNM was not on strike, if SSAUTHRAI went on strike, the nurses would also join in. This greatly empowered the Senior Staff Association, which should normally consist only of the technologists, pharmacists, and other non-medical health professionals, and made them into a potent industrial force.

The Non-Academic Staff Union of Educational and Associated Institutions (NASU) represented the non-professional staff—this meant predominantly the junior staff. They were no more militant than the other unions, but their industrial actions were really feared, because of their violence, which included a prominent use of *juju*. Apart from violence, they also used the weapon of shutting down the support services, including electricity and water supply and environmental sanitation. The only way to function if they did go on strike was that others, i.e., the health professionals, should take over their work. This was something that the union resisted violently and which only highly dedicated staff would take on, even if their lives were not threatened.

During industrial actions, we usually managed to keep essential services going, at least initially. However, if they continued for more than a week or two, strikes by the doctors and nurses, and by the Senior Staff Association, usually led to the eventual virtual shutdown of the hospital. When NASU went on strike, we could maintain essential services for longer by, as discreetly as possible, using the administrative staff, supported by those other workers who were ready to take on the risk of running the essential support services. It was under these circumstances that I learnt to run the hospital's water supply systems. I would operate the boreholes and fill the tanks first thing in the morning and last thing at night when this could be done inconspicuously. Patients' relatives would help with cleaning and took over the care of those who remained in hospital, procuring their drugs, food, and other requirements, and sometimes participating in their dressings. The operative word was "discreet." As much as possible, these operations were carried out clandestinely. If the relationship with the union was reasonably good, and it was so during my tenure, the union would turn a blind eye, since they knew these were life threatening situations.

I ran into trouble only once. In 1994, there was a protracted strike by NASU in all the nation's teaching hospitals. Since none of the other unions was involved, we managed to maintain essential services in the Ife unit. However, in the Wesley Guild Hospital, the striking workers were much more militant, and they refused to allow the wards to be cleaned. I then did a very foolish thing. I drove up to Ilesa, got hold of the Unit Administrator and the Physician-in-Charge and we started cleaning the wards, starting with the Male Medical Ward. A couple of doctors joined us. The patients and their relatives looked on aghast. We had just finished one half of the ward and started on the other when we became aware of an increasing tumult from outside—the noise of an approaching mob. Shortly thereafter, a group of about 30 men and women burst into the ward, shouting and waving sticks. The one in the forefront, who I later found was a worker from the water supply section, appeared to be particularly angry. He rushed at me and beat me on the head and body with the branch of a shrub, which was later confirmed to be *Pasan. Pasan,* also known as *atori* in Yoruba, has the botanical name *Glyphaea brevis*. The plant is attributed to have notorious magical powers. It is presumed that if anyone hits you with it, you become weak and fall to the ground. There is, at least for some, an even more sinister long-term effect: impotence! I did not fall to the ground, but was severely shaken. Dr. Agboola, one of the house officers who had been cleaning the ward with us, retaliated in my defense. There was a melée lasting about five minutes, following which the union members withdrew. However, they had achieved their aim—the hospital unit was closed down. During a subsequent investigation, we identified the *pasan* wielding individual, who, no longer supported by a mob of his colleagues, and, possibly, no longer emboldened by a good dose of Indian hemp, fainted during an identity parade. He was subsequently downgraded, but thereafter proved to be a very committed and hardworking member of the Water Unit until his retirement ten years later. We did not dismiss him, partly because of the remorse he had shown, but more importantly, because we knew he was not the real instigator of the mob. He had been merely thrust to the front, and, influenced by the law of the mob, carried out acts that he would never have committed under normal circumstances. Incidentally, if anyone is wondering whether the second potent property of *pasan* worked on me. I am glad to report that it did not!

The Wesley Guild Hospital incident is a good example of how not to manage an industrial action. In going to the hospital in broad daylight and setting about cleaning the wards, we had provoked the striking workers. We had also played into the hands of the union through an action that instigated its members, in their view, to violence. Closure of the unit was the result, which was just what the union wanted.

I have always maintained that doctors should never go on strike. I did participate in a relatively innocuous work-to-rule during my housemanship year, but since then, I have not participated in a single industrial action. However, I must admit that there is an overpowering counter-argument which is difficult to fault—strikes are the only language the Government understands. The Government really needs to treat the health profession with more responsibility. All the industrial actions that took place during my period in charge of the hospital were based on genuine grievances. They were all resolved, but why did the Government need to allow strike actions to take place before the issues were resolved?

One near disaster almost occurred during a strike by NASU in 1995. On this occasion, the security staff joined the strike, and we had to rely on a small number of local armed guards. The Children's Orthopaedic Ward in the Ife unit had recently been opened, and it was located in an otherwise undeveloped area of the hospital's premises. I gave them a walkie-talkie, and we also stationed some of the local armed guards there. At around 2am, over my walkie-talkie, I heard the nursing staff of the ward report that they were hearing gunfire from the student nurses' hostel, which was located half a kilometre away. I jumped into my car and drove from the University campus, where I lived, to the Divisional Police Headquarters in the town, where some armed policemen joined me. We drove through the hospital to the hostel. As we approached the hostel, the two armed guards stationed there came up and said that the armed robbers had attacked the hostel.The guards had retired into hiding after firing and exhausting their weapons, which were single-shot dane guns. They reported that the attack on the hostel was still going on. At this point, my police companions wanted to stop and reconnoitre. I insisted that we must go straight to the hostel. They reluctantly followed me. We found the hostel in darkness, and not a single sound coming from within it. Indeed, when we entered, we thought the hostel was deserted. Then we started hearing the sounds of frightened female voices, and the students gradually emerged from under their beds. They stated that when the robbers, numbering ten or more, heard our approach, they ran off. No one was hurt, and the robbers had not had time to steal anything. If we had arrived ten minutes later, terrible things might have happened to the unfortunate young ladies. The walkie-talkie system really saved us.

Through all the strike actions in the hospital, we never succeeded in stopping salaries. During one nation-wide crisis involving the doctors and nurses, Olikoye Ransome-Kuti issued a directive that the striking workers should not be paid. None of the teaching hospitals implemented the directive. I have to admit that I was desperate not to do anything that would provoke my colleagues further and did not for one moment consider stopping the salaries. Perhaps a desire to be in the good books of the staff, especially my own colleagues, also played a part in the decision. However, I believed then as I believe now that one answer to incessant strike actions, especially those that are irresponsible, is to implement the "No work, no pay" law. This is an internationally accepted principle, and, to my knowledge, only in Nigeria do individuals abandon their duties and still expect to be paid. By not implementing the principle, strike actions become virtually paid holidays.

V

Development and other Initiatives

¤ ¤ ¤ ¤ ¤ ¤ ¤ ¤ ¤ ¤ ¤ ¤

During an accreditation visit to our postgraduate programme in Internal Medicine by the National Postgraduate Medical College, the leader of the team asked me about the institution's developmental plan. Hesitantly, I mentioned that we wanted to develop our Renal Programme. At that point, I realised that we did not have a Development Plan. We only had a list of capital projects that we considered priorities. Prior to that time, we had been concentrating on providing the basic services required for the hospital to function properly, i.e., infrastructural rehabilitation, supplies of medicines and consumables, the efficiency of emergency care, etc. These priorities were not formally documented. We carried out development on an ad-hoc basis. For example, we decided early on that we should embark on a programme of training the various specialists that we needed and just got on with this. We did not budget for this project properly and were lucky that we were able to fund such training from a broad vote head for staff training. As another example, when we decided that the mortuary services in the Wesley Guild Hospital Unit were inadequate, we simply embarked on a project to expand the mortuary and install a new refrigeration system there. We never actually planned for this initially.

Individual departments had their priorities, and put them forward. If the Administration liked an idea, we just went for it. This lack of a development plan could have been disastrous. What perhaps saved the situation was that, for much of the time, we concentrated on developing and improving basic services. Even though we did not have a documented development plan, we had a basic one in our minds, or, at least, I did. It must be emphasised that a documented development plan is essential for any organization so everyone concerned can be aware of the priorities of the organisation, and of their place and role in it. Coordinated development is impossible without a plan and it is also important for budgeting purposes.

One major reason why we did not have a plan was that I had no management training. I came into the administration of the institution without experience or training in administration. When, towards the end of my job as CMD, I was exposed to some short management courses, my eyes were truly opened. I believe that any doctor who wishes to go into management should have proper training in Health Care and Hospital Management. When I was in charge of the hospital, the majority of CMDs in the country were in the same position as I was. Their only qualification to administer their institutions was that they were medical specialists. We had to learn on the job, supplemented by the occasional short courses organised by the Ministry of Health or, in one instance, the World Bank. It is unfortunate that many of my colleagues in the medical profession still do not accept that medical administrators need to have management training.

The Renal Programme was one of our major developments. This programme actually had its origins in the 1970s, when the wife of a prominent academic in the University died of kidney failure. The academic challenged the Faculty (it was then a Faculty) of Health Sciences to develop facilities for the management of renal disease and even provided some funds for this. The initial, tentative steps did not yield much progress, but the seed had been planted. During my predecessor's term, a Haemodialysis Unit was developed. This was commissioned in November 1987, soon after I was appointed Acting CMD. Dr. (now Professor) Wale Akinsola was the leader of the Renal Team. I worked closely with him. The objective was to develop a comprehensive renal service comprising:

- A community-based programme of prevention and early diagnosis and treatment of renal disease and its causes.
- Dialysis services, comprising haemodialysis services and Continuous Ambulatory Peritoneal Dialysis (CAPD) services. CAPD involves continuous infusion of the abdominal cavity with fluids which extract the waste products that are normally removed by the kidneys.
- Kidney transplantation.

An abandoned building project, originally proposed as an amenity ward, was modified and completed as a renal ward. Dr. Okechukwu Onuzo, who had a haemodialysis service in Lagos, gave extremely valuable technical advice and support. A programme of staff training and technical cooperation was started with the University of Manchester's Renal Team. Very soon, the institutions' renal programme became renowned for the quality of its service. Wale Akinsola and his team must take the credit for this—they were highly committed, and highly skilled. Sister Eunice Akoma, the senior nurse in charge of the unit, must also be specially mentioned. The haemodialysis service functioned efficiently until I left office. We had a technical agent, Mr. O.P. Asika, who, against many odds, always managed to keep the machines working.

The CAPD service was not successful. The fluids had to be imported from abroad, as local manufacturers could not make them. On one occasion when we imported a large batch of the fluids, an officer in the Stores Department conspired with a clearing agent to defraud the institution, and by the time the problem was sorted out, the fluids had expired. We did get a few patients started on CAPD, but the results were poor. There was a high rate of infection. One individual, presumably believing that if clear fluids were good then milk would be better, filled his CAPD bag with evaporated milk!

Through our arrangements with Manchester, and susequently with the University of Cairo, we trained nephrologists, surgeons, nurses, and an immunologist. By the end of 1996, we believed we were ready for a live donor transplant. All we needed was a new haemodialysis machine to back up the transplant in the post-operative period. As a result of the conduct of the then Minister of Health, we could not obtain the equipment and the operation was delayed. However, the delay turned out to be fortuitous. The team was probably much better prepared by the time the first transplant was carried out in 2003. The hospital's renal team is still in the forefront of that discipline. It has also provided technical support and indeed personnel, to other institutions. The hospital made history by being the first Nigerian public hospital to introduce haemodialysis and also the first to carry out kidney transplantation. The efforts of Wale Akinsola and his team show how much can be achieved by dedicated individuals, even when the resources are limited.

A substantial number of major physical projects were embarked on and completed during the Abiola-Oshodi Board's tenure. The awards were made with absolute integrity. Unfortunately, this did not stop some unscrupulous members of staff from acting against the interest of the hospital. However, the majority of members of staff were honest, dedicated and committed. We were able to get the best value for our money, because contractors did not have to give bribes or kickbacks, and knew they would be paid promptly. We made sure that no contract was awarded unless we actually had the money, thus increasing the confidence of contractors and avoiding the risk of abandoned projects. The project that gave me most personal satisfaction was the Ilesa Water Project mentioned earlier.

In 1989, many of the specialties were understaffed. The emphasis in the past had been to recruit specialists to fill these areas of need. This policy did not solve the problem. Other institutions such as the University College Hospital (UCH), Ibadan and the Lagos University Teaching Hospital

(LUTH), were more attractive to these greatly sought-after individuals. We decided that the best way forward was to embark on a programme of in-service training of specialists, focusing particularly on Ife graduates. The major advantages of this policy were that such individuals would tend to be more loyal to their alma mater proudly called "Great Ife," and with justification, and also that we could ensure that the training we sponsored was of a very high standard. We sent them mainly to the UCH and LUTH, supplemented in some cases by overseas placements. After I left office, a number were trained in South Africa. The process took many years and it involved a great financial investment. The result was that we were able to field specialists in all areas, including the rarer sub-specialties. We were also able to recruit a few specialists, including a truly dedicated and highly skilled anaesthesiologist in the person of Dr. Fola Faponle. The hospital currently has specialists in almost every major area of specialisation, and they are of the highest standard. They can stand shoulder-to-shoulder with specialists in any part of the world.

The activities of the OAUTHC extended into the community. One major project that we were involved in was the Baby Friendly Initiative (BFI). Its official title is the Baby Friendly Hospital Initiative (BFHI), but I dropped the word "Hospital" because I believe the Initiative concerns the whole community and not just hospitals.

Sometime in mid-1991, all CMDs were summoned to a meeting in Lagos by Olikoye Ransome-Kuti. He personally briefed us on the Initiative, which had as its objective the implementation of appropriate breastfeeding practices. The Initiative was a world-wide one, and incidentally, Olikoye was Chairman of the Working Party of UNICEF and WHO at which the policy had been formulated and from which the Innocenti Declaration concerning the Initiative was issued. The Declaration is named after the building, the Spegale del Innocenti in Florence, where the Working Party meeting took place. The Initiative was to cover the whole country. It was to be implemented first in the teaching hospitals and subsequently, with the experience and expertise gained, the teaching hospitals were to promote its implementation throughout the health care system and into the community. I embraced Olikoye's directive wholeheartedly, and returned to Ife full of enthusiasm. I have to admit that part of my enthusiasm was simply my confidence in Olikoye as someone who could do no wrong. However, as I came to understand the potential impact of the BFI on the health of the nation and the other benefits, I became truly dedicated to the cause. Dr. (now Professor) Friday Okonofua, then Head of the Department of Obstetrics and Gynaecology, had attended the meeting with me. On our return, we mobilised a team of like-minded individuals to get the initiative started in the institution. Apart from Friday, there was Dr. A.R. Abejide, then a senior resident; Mrs. D.E. Babajide, an experienced nurse who could "bring milk out of a stone" (she could help any mother to breastfeed successfully and was also an expert at restoring lactation if this had ceased); Mrs. Betty Owosho, another experienced nurse; Dr. Anita Davis-Adetugbo, a resident in Community Health; and Dr. Ebun Adejuyigbe, then a senior resident in paediatrics. Dr. Adejuyigbe was a great advocate of the programme as she breastfed her baby exclusively for six months during this period. We were subsequently joined by other health professionals as well as some members of the community, prominent among whom was Mrs. Moni Omole, the wife of our benefactor, Lawrence Omole.

The objectives of the BFI were:

- Exclusive breastfeeding of babies for the first six months of life.
- Continuation of breastfeeding, complemented by other (locally available) foods until the child was two years old.

This latter objective is somewhat flexible; in practice, after the first six months of exclusive breastfeeding, we encouraged breastfeeding for as long as possible, rather than rigidly advocating breastfeeding until the child was two years old. The benefits of these appropriate breastfeeding practices are substantial. They include:

- Nutritional benefits—human breast milk is ideally formulated for the growth and development of the human child, including its intellectual development.
- Human breast milk contains a number of factors which protect the baby against infections. It is actually the first immunisation that the child has. These protective factors are highly concentrated in colostrum, the first watery yellow milk that is produced by the mother in the first few days after delivery.
- The promotion of mother–child bonding, important for the psychological development of the child.
- Economic advantages as it saves on the purchase of baby formula.

Implementing the BFI involved the training of health personnel and community members and the provision of practical requirements. The orientation of health personnel and community members was also critical. It was a major task, but we made rapid progress. We also led the way. We developed the Breastfeeding Policy that was adopted by many other institutions. A year after Olikoye Ransome-Kuti held his meeting with us, the hospital was one of the four teaching hospitals that was officially designated "Baby Friendly" by UNICEF. The reward was a certificate and a Toyota Land Cruiser to assist us in the further propagation of the BFI. I collected both the certificate and the Land Cruiser at a ceremony in Ibadan and personally drove the vehicle back to Ife in triumph.

We took the work in earnest, by implementing the BFI throughout Osun State. Since, at least within the "orthodox" health care system, most antenatal care and the delivery of the majority of babies took place in the Primary Health Care (PHC) system, we decided that our efforts should be focused on that system, which is under local governments. The first Local Government Area to show an interest was Irepodun, with its headquarters in Ilobu. We became aware of this interest when the PHC coordinator, Mr. M.B. Segilola, requested that we should assist the Local Government to develop baby friendly facilities. I suspect that part of their motivation was the desire to win a Toyota Land Cruiser. However, even when it became obvious that such a vehicle was unlikely to materialise, they still embarked on the project enthusiastically. The Chairman of the Local Government, Chief Emmanuel Oyedeji, was totally committed to the programme. We organised training for all the PHC personnel, and worked with them to make their health centres baby friendly. We developed a Breastfeeding Policy specifically for PHC facilities which they could adapt to their needs. We also developed one for secondary care facilities. In less than a year, the facilities were inspected and all eight health centres were designated Baby Friendly by UNICEF. From there on, things really took off. Other local governments, wanting to emulate the success of Irepodun, joined the bandwagon. Most of the local governments had their facilities designated baby friendly. Local governments deal directly with the community, and it was relatively easy to involve communities, who readily accepted and joined in the programme.

I was appointed Coordinator for B-Zone (South-West Nigeria) in 1992, and the team worked with all the seven states in the zone. Osun State was repeatedly declared the leading baby friendly state in successive years and B-zone the leading zone. The other states in the zone were not far behind. The BFI made a major impact all over the country. More and more families adopted the appropriate breastfeeding practices. Prior to the initiative, the majority of babies were breastfed. However, exclusive breastfeeding was rare and the duration of breastfeeding was variable. Community surveys indicated a substantial success of the programme and of its benefits.

In 1987, UNICEF appointed a new Representative in Nigeria. With his arrival, things began to change. UNICEF, in consultation with the Federal Ministry of Health, decided that it would promote a new, expanded, initiative termed the "Mother and Child Friendly Initiative", which would promote the provision of a number of essential services for mothers and babies. The BFI was to be absorbed into this new initiative. Support was virtually withdrawn for the BFI while the new initiative was supposedly being implemented.

The new initiative did not take off. I regret that the practices in breastfeeding are gradually reverting to the old ways. Exclusive breastfeeding is declining, and more and more children are being bottle-fed, either partly or completely. Of course, a major aspect of the problem was the failure to build sustainability into the programme. This is one of the problems with such programmes. Initiatives come and go, and often do not have enduring effects because strategies are not built into them towards their sustainability. I believe we should have been making efforts to promote sustained changes in knowledge and beliefs through the educational system for health professionals as well as through the general educational system. I stated this repeatedly, but the powers that be did not take the necessary action. One exception is the training programmes for nurses and midwives, into which the BFI has been successfully integrated.

VI

Community Crises

⌗ ⌗ ⌗ ⌗ ⌗ ⌗ ⌗ ⌗ ⌗ ⌗ ⌗

There are two major communal groups within Ile-Ife. According to Yoruba folklore, Ile-Ife is the place where the human race was established. If you do not believe this, I can take you to the site in the centre of the city where *Oduduwa* came down from heaven and established the human race! If you do not believe that story, then at least we know that the city dates back to the Eleventh Century or earlier, and that *Oduduwa* was probably the first major leader of the people who today call themselves the Ifes. A substantial number of other Yoruba cities and towns were subsequently established by migrants from Ile-Ife, many of them by the children of *Oduduwa*. Thus, Ife and its people date back many centuries, and its traditional ruler, the *Ooni*, is, arguably, the most prominent of the Yoruba rulers.

Following the fall of the Old Oyo Empire in the 1830s, a large group of displaced people arrived in Ife and settled in the city. Subsequently, because of problems between the newcomers and the Ifes, the *Ooni* allowed the newcomers to settle in a separate nearby area to the west, now called Modakeke. This action by the *Ooni* greatly angered his people, and resulted in the death of the monarch. Some of the people originally displaced from the Old Oyo Empire also settled in some other neighbouring areas, and are generally regarded as allied to the Modakekes. As both the original Ile-Ife and the settlement at Modakeke expanded, their boundaries merged. However, the Ifes have continued to claim that the Modakekes do not own the territory on which they live, but are merely tenants who were allowed to settle on it. On the other hand, the Modakekes claim sovereignty over the territory that they occupy. The two opposing stances are an obvious prescription for conflict and for almost two centuries there have been problems between the two communities. During the wars of the Nineteenth Century in Yorubaland, the Modakekes sided with the Ibadans against Ife and its allies, and on two occasions, aided the Ibadan army in sacking Ile-Ife. Wars between the two communities have erupted from time to time since then.

In August 1997, the conflict flared up again. The two communities armed themselves and literally went to war. The warriors on both sides were armed with guns as well as swords and machetes, reinforced by numerous charms meant to protect them against the other force's weapons, including bullets. There were regular gun battles, mainly at the boundaries of the two communities. However, no area was safe, because there were frequent forays by the two warring factions into each other's territories. Large numbers of casualties poured into the Accidents and Emergencies Department of the Ife State Hospital, and the staff worked day and night. The hospital was full of gunshot victims and victims with horrific knife and machete wounds. We had just acquired a Computer Tomographic Scanner, which was invaluable in the investigations of the injuries. This equipment became so heavily used that on one occasion it shut down, signaling that it had been exposed to an excessive amount of metal. These were the bullets from the casualties.

The Blood Bank soon ran out, and we also ran out of volunteer donors. Early one night, I went to the *Aafin* (the *Ooni*'s palace). There was a huge crowd of armed men guarding the *Aafin*. Fortunately they recognised me, or I would have been in grave danger. At that time, members of the two communities who strayed into the other's territory were being kidnapped, taken to an area set aside for the purpose and killed. Although I explained that I wanted an audience with the *Ooni*, I was not allowed into his presence but was handed a telephone over which I discussed the situation with him. Having explained the steps we had taken to treat the wounded, I requested for blood donors. He promised that volunteers would show up the following day, and they did.

The Ife State Hospital, and indeed, our other facility in the town, the Urban Comprehensive Health Centre, was in Ife territory. Although we had members of staff from both communities, the Ifes were well in the majority. As soon as the crisis erupted, the staff from Modakeke ran for their lives and most did not come back until several years later. The majority of staff from Modakeke had to be deployed to Ilesa, where many of them remain till today. Only Ifes and those considered to be their allies were able to receive treatment in the hospital during the crisis. The Modakekes and individuals from communities considered by the Ifes to be allied to them had to seek treatment elsewhere. Indeed, I still see some people from Modakeke in my Psychiatry clinic in Ilesa. They still feel endangered going to the Ife State Hospital, where we also have a psychiatric unit. I felt proud of the manner in which the hospital treated many of the casualties, but also felt ashamed at the manner in which the staff had actively rejected the Modakekes. Soon after the conflict erupted, some members of staff conspired to stop the salaries of the members of staff from Modakeke. We detected this in the nick of time, and I had to personally supervise the final processing of salaries to ensure that everyone was paid.

The Ifes had two great "warriors" — "Apollo" and "Yellow" — the latter was so named because of his light complexion. They were renowned for their leadership, courage and ability in combat. Yellow was brought into the Accidents and Emergencies Department with multiple wounds. He was literally covered with charms. Unfortunately, he was dead on arrival. Some days after that, Apollo, also bedecked with charms, was brought in with multiple wounds; he was gasping, and all efforts to resuscitate him failed. He was the Number One "warrior" and there was grief all over the town. The following morning, as I was driving to work, I noticed numerous people jubilating. I could not hear what they were saying, but was later told it was Apollo *ti dide* ("Apollo has risen up" [from the dead]). Apparently, the medicine man who had furnished Apollo with the charms had given an assurance that he had taken the necessary steps to revive him. The *Ooni* was presented with the news of Apollo's revival and sent one of his high chiefs to check. In the mortuary, I found that Apollo was still dead. When I told the high chief, he burst into tears.

Charms were the order of the day during this conflict, and indeed the subsequent "war" a decade later. It was tragic to see so many young people being brought into Casualty seriously wounded, taking their last breath or dead on arrival. All were literally covered in charms. They all truly believed that the charms would protect them even from bullets.

Charms and other paraphernalia of "native medicine" or *oogun* feature prominently in this book. I humourously employ the term *juju*. As the reader will observe from the subsequent sections dealing with my period as chief executive of the University, the belief in this phenomenon stretches across the entire community. Even people with PhDs have a great fear of *juju*, and will resort to its use when circumstances dictate. I have earlier related the incident when I was assaulted with *pasan* during an industrial crisis, fortunately with no ill effects. On the other hand, on a number of occasions I saw members of staff who, having been struck by rings or other implements that had been given magical treatment, became absolutely terrified over prospects of their impending demise.

One serious event involving a claim of malignant use of *oogun* did occur in 1990—the *moko moko* episode. The term means "robbing men of their penises." Around that time, there was a rumour going round Ilesa that some individuals were taking away men's genitals for use in preparing a potent medicine for making money. One morning, in the School of Nursing in the Wesley Guild Hospital, a 17-year old male student nurse suddenly shouted out that his penis had disappeared, and went into a panic. His colleagues, both male and female, immediately believed him, and there was uproar while they started looking for the perpetrator. A young man, who had been sent on an errand to the hospital by his mother, was walking outside the school at the time and was apprehended. He was recognised as the son of the proprietor of the *Iyadunni* Restaurant, the most popular eating place in the town. *Iyadunni* was the subject of much envy among other individuals in the restaurant trade, and, as is our custom, it was assumed that she employed supernatural means to make her food delicious and attract customers. The crowd of young students became convinced that the young man had been sent to the hospital by his mother to steal a penis which was to be the ingredient in a potion. They grabbed him and beat him mercilessly. Some of them, including a male and a female student whom we later identified, then started torturing him in a truly gruesome manner in order to extract a confession.

The Principal of the school and some of his teachers intervened, and were initially able to restore some order. The students insisted that their colleague's penis had truly been removed. A female nurse tutor volunteered to examine the young man and to confirm whether his penis had actually been removed. She retired into a room with the student and returned to announce, "His penis is still there but it is smaller than usual!" The student nurses were incensed by this news and resumed their frenzied attack on the unfortunate young man. The Principal, aided by some other tutors, managed to smuggle him out, at the cost of serious injuries to the Principal.

The story went round the entire town. Many people believed that the phallic loss had actually occurred, and for some months, *Iyadunni*'s clientele greatly reduced. We set up an enquiry which was able to identify the major culprits. I expelled them, but they subsequently went to court and obtained injunctions against my actions. Eventually, the Board of Management changed their punishments to suspensions, and I believe most of them, including the young man whose penis had either disappeared or diminished in size, eventually finished their training. I wonder what they would feel about the episode today, if they were to reflect on it. I now believe my punishment of dismissal was excessively harsh, but I was truly incensed by the way they had tortured the unfortunate young man. However, this was really a case of mass hysteria, compounded by the law of the mob.

VII

Time Out

⌸ ⌸ ⌸ ⌸ ⌸ ⌸ ⌸ ⌸ ⌸ ⌸ ⌸

The hospital was hard work for me. I was extremely busy for most days and most nights. However, I tried to keep free the period from around 2pm on Saturday and the whole of Sunday. My wife, Dorothy, was working in Saudi Arabia, but my two sons, Roger and Tony, were with me. We lived in a bungalow on the University campus. I did the cooking, but an indispensable lady named Grace Odere, who has been with us since 1988, did the cleaning and laundry twice a week. Roger and Tony attended Moremi High School on the campus. At that time, Moremi High School was one of the best secondary schools in the country. The Principal, Mr. J.A. Ogunwuyi, was a dedicated and capable individual, and he had some equally committed and capable teachers. Later on, both my sons gained admission into the University. My late hours left me with relatively little time with the two boys during the week, but I tried to make up for it at weekends.

As they grew up, they developed their own circles of friends, so that the activities in which we used to participate jointly, especially fishing, began to attract less of their interest. Indeed, I believe that I did not give them enough attention.

My main interest was fishing. Every Sunday, after the early morning service at the All Souls Chapel on the University campus, I would go off with my close friend Olu Arigbabu and another friend, Leo Dare, either to the main reservoir on the campus or to one of the reservoirs on the Agricultural Farm. Olu Arigbabu, a surgeon, and I have been friends since I came to Ile-Ife in 1978 — a friendship which blossomed primarily because of our joint interest in fishing. He also shared my interests in some other activities, especially beer. Leo is a Professor of Political Science, now living in Canada. He was the most proficient angler of the three of us, and also had an uncanny ability to detect the whereabouts of the bait we most commonly employed — a species of large, tough worms. His stock of scurrilous stories was inexhaustible, and he would constantly have us in fits of laughter. After each session, we would retire to one of our homes and sit out in the garden, drinking beer. It was idyllic, and it still is.

My second hobby was cricket. In the 1980s, a staff cricket team was formed following a discussion in the Staff Club. Our first match was against our children in Moremi High School, but subsequently we played against teams from Ibadan and Lagos, and, of course, the University's student team. It was cricket that cemented my friendship with a number of individuals and their families: Akin Aboderin, the skipper of the team, 'Lanre Togonu-Bickersteth, a prolific batsman, and Bayo Amole, a truly fast bowler, who designed the house I am still building in the town. I had known Vince Nwuga for quite a long time before, and he became our "No nonsense" umpire. Vince had a particular habit of going off "to town" after every session. There were about 15 of us, and we had a great time, not just from cricket, but from the truly enjoyable social life that was built around the game.

There is one other couple I must mention — Professor David Ijalaye and Mrs. Joke Ijalaye. They were among the first friends we made after we arrived in Ife in 1978 and we regard both of them as family. Both of them are, of course, much older than us and we call them Uncle David and Aunty Joke. They have been our greatest source of support and advice. Throughout the period I served in the hospital, and also throughout my subsequent term in the University as Vice Chancellor, Uncle David was my chief adviser and confidant. How great it is to have people like them who are always there for you, and whom you can trust completely.

Dorothy was working in Saudi Arabia for two reasons. First, someone had to make some money. Also, as a radiologist, she had the facilities over there with which she could meaningfully apply her skills. She came over twice a year and I also went over there less frequently. When we were together, things were just great. When she wasn't around, I was content in the knowledge that I had her full support in the work I was doing. In fact, if she had been living with me in Ife, our marriage might have run into trouble because of my rather excessively long working hours.

I have always stuck to a very limited number of friends. Indeed, I am a bit of a loner. I enjoy being with people I trust and who share my interests. I also quite enjoy sitting on my own in the garden on an evening, drinking beer and reading a book or watching the sunset. One other source of relaxation I have is walking, particularly on the three hills on the University campus. I regularly climbed the hills with Roger and Tony, and after their interests were diverted to other things, I still climbed the hills alone. There is nothing quite as enjoyable as walking through our beautiful campus. This will be addressed in more detail later on, but this issue is raised now because the campus means so much to me. The campus is what kept me sane in the high pressure job of the CMD. More and more people have taken up walking and jogging round the campus in recent years, but at that time only a few would consider going anywhere except in their cars.

I truly enjoyed walking. During one three-week period of a national strike, which was compounded by a severe fuel shortage, I took to walking to work. The distance involved was about seven kilometres. I would leave my house on the University campus at about 6.00 am in the morning, and arrive around 7.30 am. I truly enjoyed the walk, and found a number of paths and minor roads which avoided the main roads. Coming back was more difficult because of the heat, but I still enjoyed it. I was setting an example, but it was no real effort on my part; rather, it was truly pleasurable. From time to time, taxi drivers would offer to give me lifts, free of charge. They must have thought it was my pride that made me refuse; it was not. Some others must have thought I was a mad *Oyinbo* (white man). After all, Noel Coward did write that only mad dogs and Englishmen go out into the midday sun, a concept very familiar to the Yoruba people who believe that the "hot" deity *Sonponna* is more likely to be encountered in the heat of the afternoon! Meetings with Sonponna are believed to be one cause of madness.

VIII

End of Term

ⅹ ⅹ ⅹ ⅹ ⅹ ⅹ ⅹ ⅹ ⅹ ⅹ

My second term as Chief Medical Director ended on 16 November 1997. At that time, we did not have a Board of Management. I knew that there was some campaigning going on for the new appointment. It was clear that my successor would not be appointed in time for me to personally hand over to him. When asked in the Ministry who should be appointed Acting CMD, I suggested that the Chairman, Medical Advisory Committee, Dr. David Akinola, be given this temporary appointment. As recorded earlier, David remained a very capable, committed, and loyal individual who had the advantage of having worked closely with me for two years. By the time I left, his letter of appointment had not come through, so I had to write a letter asking him to look after the institution until his letter arrived from the Ministry. David Akinola was eventually appointed substantive CMD to my great delight. I was truly delighted to preside over the meeting of the University's Appointments and Promotions Committee where his promotion as Professor was approved in 2000.

I refused an official "send-off" ceremony by the hospital, but a small group of my closest associates, calling themselves the Committee of Friends, insisted on organising one. I had expected a low key affair, but several hundred members of staff and well-wishers attended the event. I gave a "valedictory" lecture, following which there was a huge luncheon party. How this small group of friends could afford such largesse I do not know.They must have taxed themselves heavily to throw the party. The huge number of well-wishers who attended the event included Dr. Abiola-Oshodi and Dr. Toyosi. Even the Ooni was represented by some of his high chiefs. There was speech after speech, praising me to high heavens. I hope they truly meant it! At one point, members of NASU carried me aloft along the corridors, singing my praises. I believe the majority of the members of staff valued my contribution to the hospital and to their welfare. Even now, over ten years afterwards, I still get an enthusiastic welcome from them wherever I go to the hospital. However, the Government never acknowledged the work I did, and the progress that the institution recorded during my eight plus years in charge. There is just one sign in the hospital that I was ever CMD—the low lift pump house of the Wesley Guild Hospital water works has an inscription on it saying "Professor R.O.A. Makanjuola Dam." Whenever the paint fades, I beg the maintenance officer in charge to repaint this sign!

The day after the send-off party, I undertook the important but sad official task of handing over the body of the late Chief AdekunleAjasin to the Osun State Military Governor, Colonel Nwosu, at the start of the late chief's final journey to his home town, Owo. The day after that, I handed over the hospital to David Akinola and travelled to The Gambia for the Annual General and Scientific Meeting of the West African College of Physicians.

Thus ended my first foray into administration.

Two questions arise. First, did I make a difference to the hospital? An objective answer can only be provided by an impartial observer, and not by the central figure. However, I believe that I did make a difference. The hospital was certainly a better place when I left it than when I arrived. This is my opinion.

I am sure there will be those, perhaps many, who will disagree with this self-assessment.

A more cogent question would concern the new system of administering the teaching hospitals, which has been adopted for most specialist and even many general hospitals in Nigeria. I believe I am in a specially advantaged position to provide an opinion on this. I spent over eight years as Chief Executive between 1989 and 1997. During the ten months that I served as Acting CMD from September 1984 to July 1985, I was also the first of the new cadre of full-time CMDs. During that period, although I was being paid by the University, I did the job more or less full-time, while the old system of Deans as CMDs continued in other teaching institutions. I was thus the first true full-time medical chief executive of a teaching hospital.

In most parts of the world, the recent trend has been to place the administration of health care facilities in the hands of a new breed of professionals called Health Care Managers. These individuals undergo degree courses in the discipline. Medical administrators (i.e. doctors and dentists) continue to function in this new system, but their role is restricted to purely clinical matters and the real power lies in the hands of the new breed of health care administrators. This was the trend in Nigerian teaching hospitals until the promulgation of Decree No. 10 of 1985. Why are we different?

A number of arguments have been put forward in favour of the new system of administration. First, only a small proportion of health care administration concerns strictly medical matters. When I was CMD, much of the work consisted of ensuring the supply of water and electricity, maintenance of facilities, hospital sanitation, stores and pharmacy supplies, personnel matters, and the like. Why should medical professionals spend so much of their time on such matters? One could argue that medical doctors have unique knowledge and skills which are so valuable that their time should be spent exercising that knowledge and those skills. To put it bluntly, what is our business looking after the cleaning of the hospital when we should be in the operating theatre? Most importantly, doctors and dentists do not have expertise in management. Their medical training does not include this discipline.

The major arguments in favour of doctors as managers are mainly advanced by the members of the medical profession. They argue that doctors and dentists have a comprehensive knowledge of health care, and are therefore in the best position to manage the system. Also, by dint of the length and nature of their training, which is greater than that of any other health professional, doctors and dentists should be the bosses and should not be subservient to anyone. I would add that we hold on to the traditional belief that doctors are superior beings who know everything there is to know about health care, including administration. A medical colleague once put this very succinctly "I am a doctor; why should I need management training?" We all tend to believe we are superior to all other beings, including the other health professionals, and certainly far superior to the "bloody administrators."

The other health professionals are actually arguing that any health professional should be capable of administering the hospital system, and are clamouring for equal opportunities in this regard. They argue that they have just as much knowledge and skills in hospital administration as the medical profession. If they do get their way, which seems rather unlikely in view of the political climate, then one wonders what their titles will be: "Chief Nursing Director?", "Chief Medical Laboratory Technologist Director"?, "Chief Environmental Health Director?" of the hospital?

And the hospital administrators, who believe they have been robbed of their positions, are standing by, and perhaps, also scheming for the return to the good old days!

The arguments go back and forth. However, there is an important question that must be asked: Has the health care system been better managed since doctors assumed or regained control? I am not sure that we have an answer to that question.

In the late 1980s and 1990s, most of us learnt on the job. However, such learning takes time and may also be defective in some areas. Much of what I learnt on the job is taught in health management programmes. The few short courses that I attended were eye-openers. However, it would be far better if doctors were exposed to the required training before they start to administer the system, or at least early in their period of duty. I firmly believe that instruction in management should be included in the curricula of medical and dental training, especially at the postgraduate level. The West African College of Physicians, and, I believe, the National Postgraduate Medical College of Nigeria, do organise such courses, but they are of limited scope. The doctor who wants to go into central administration should undergo more comprehensive management training, for example the three-month certificate or the twelve-month diploma course in Health Administration organised by universities and institutes of administration.

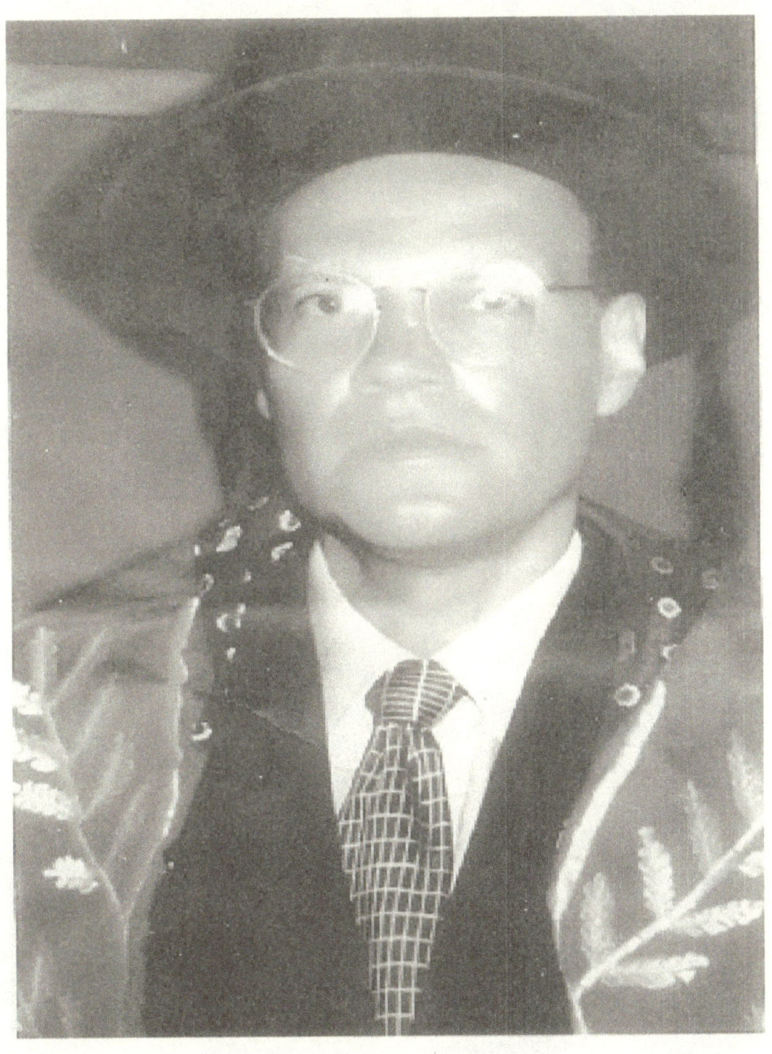

Author
(Professor Roger Makanjuola)

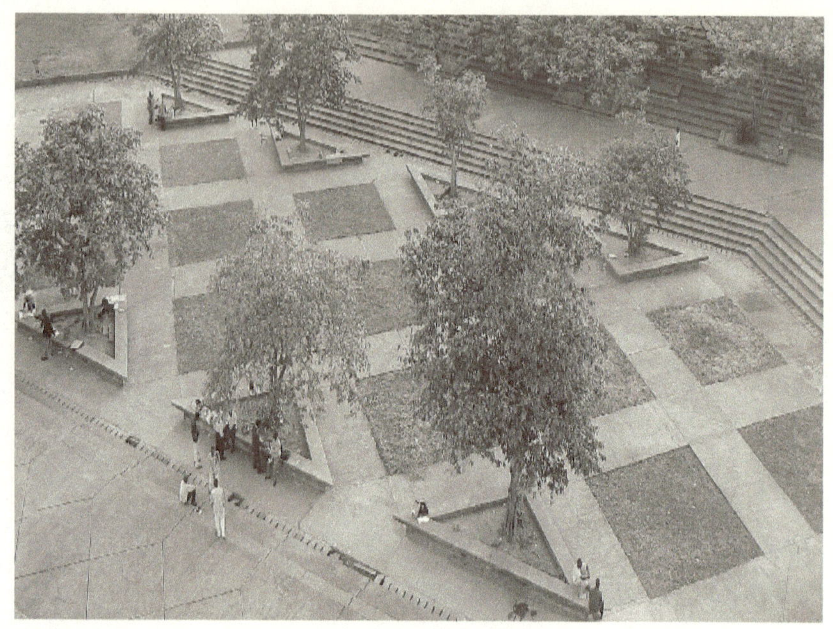

Our beautiful campus

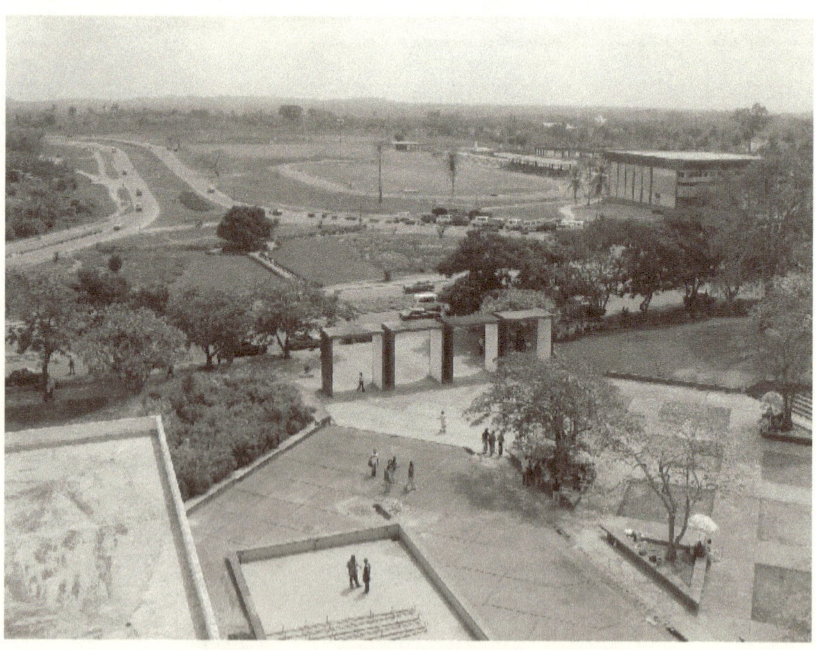

The Sports Centre and Motion Ground

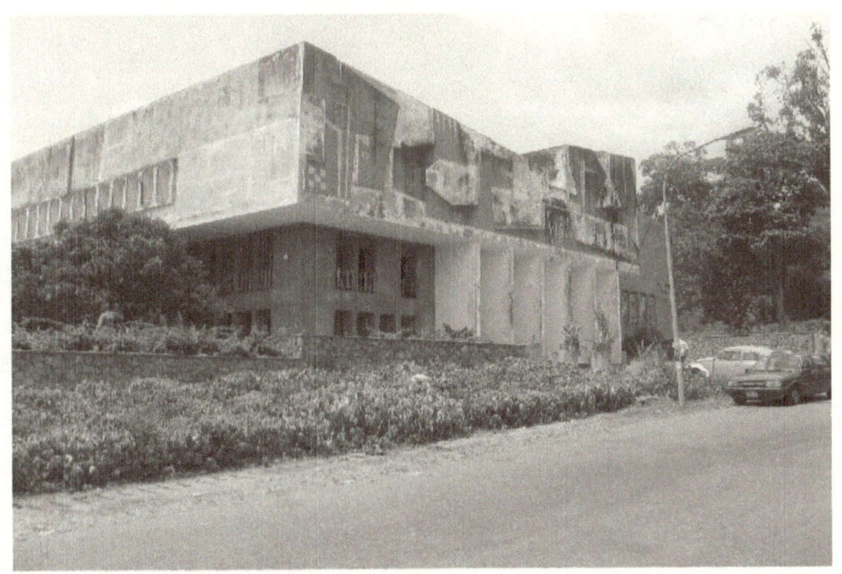

The African Studies Building before renovation

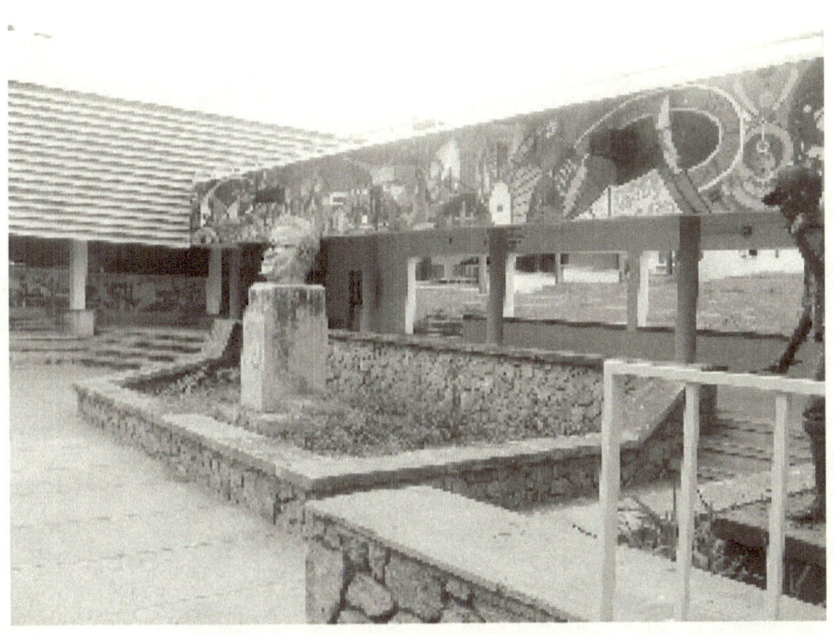

The African Studies Building after renovation

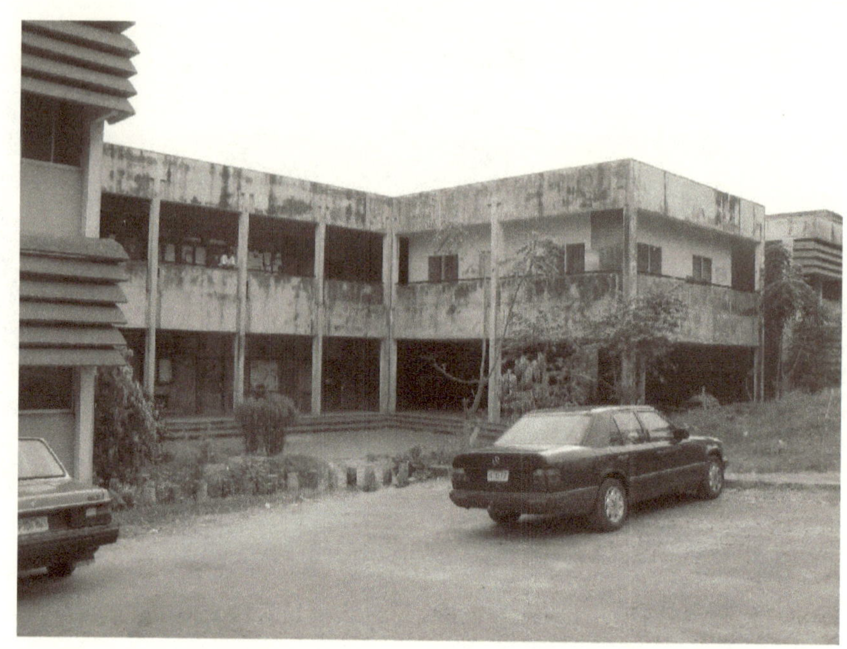

The Biological Sciences Building before renovation

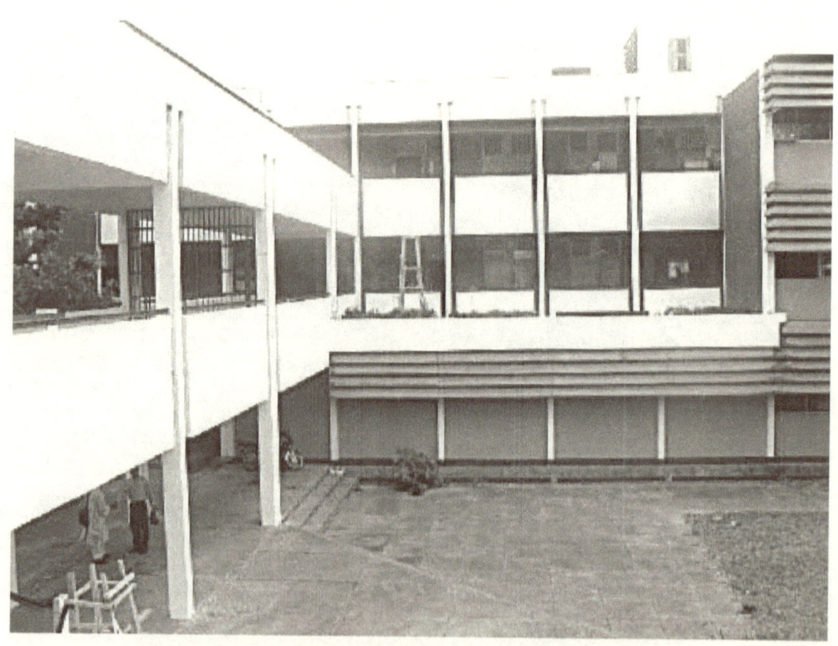

The Biological Sciences Building after renovation

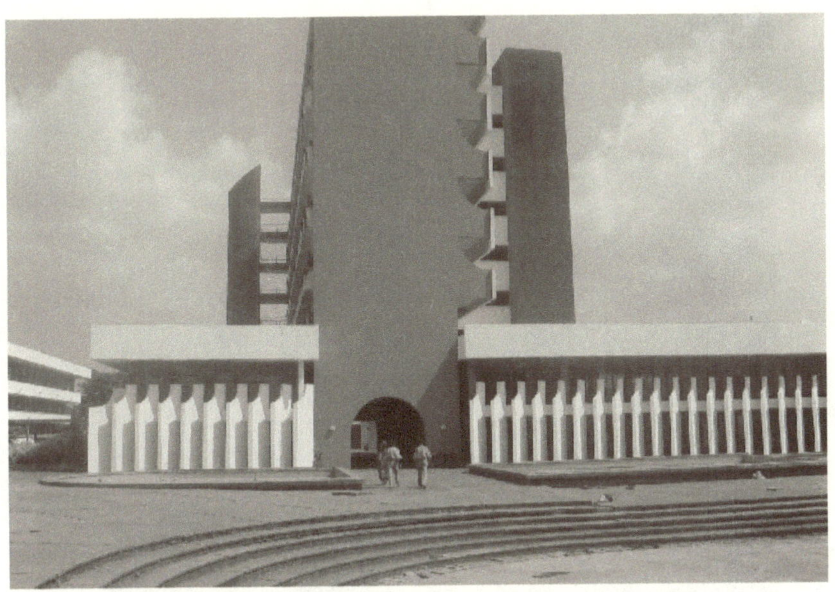

The OAU Renovation Project—The University Hall

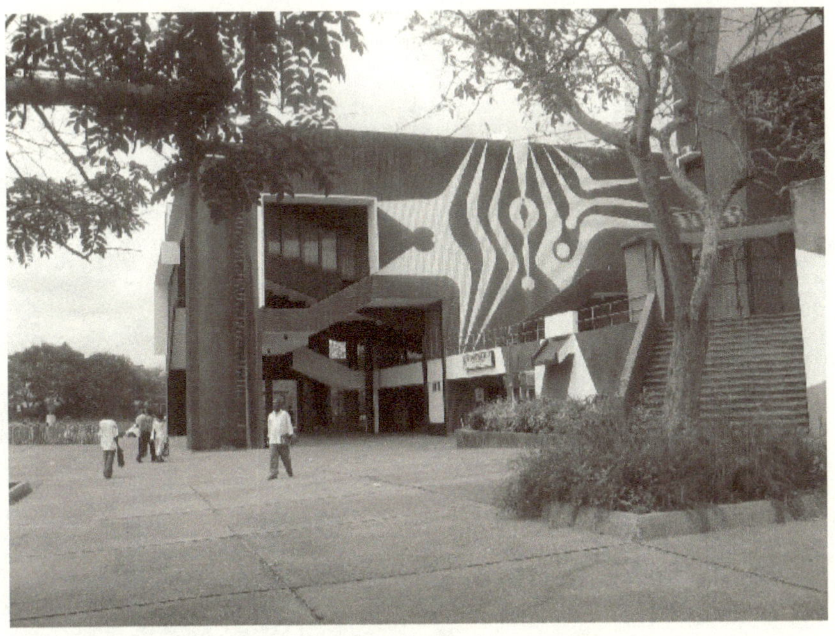

The OAU Renovation Project—Oduduwa Hall

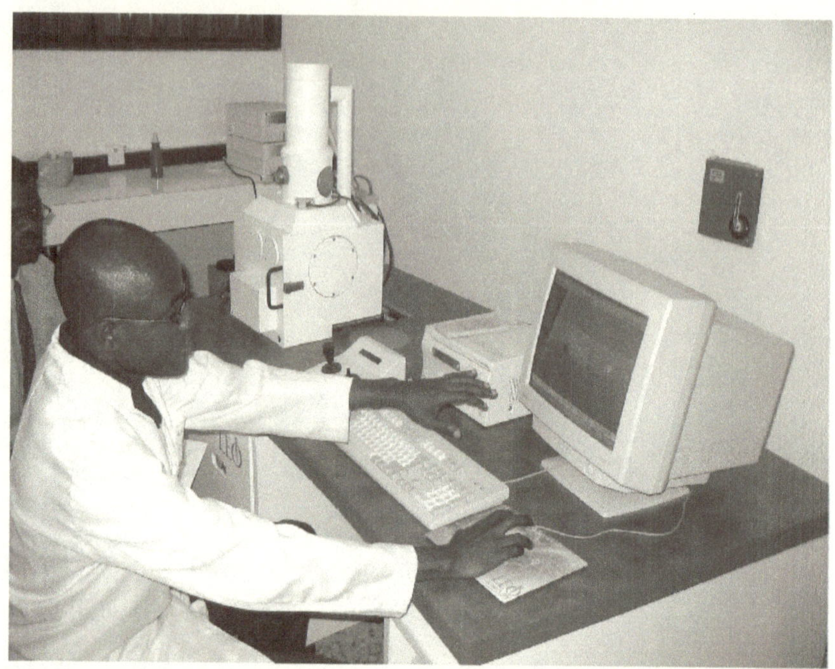

The Central Science Laboratory—Scanning Electron Microscope

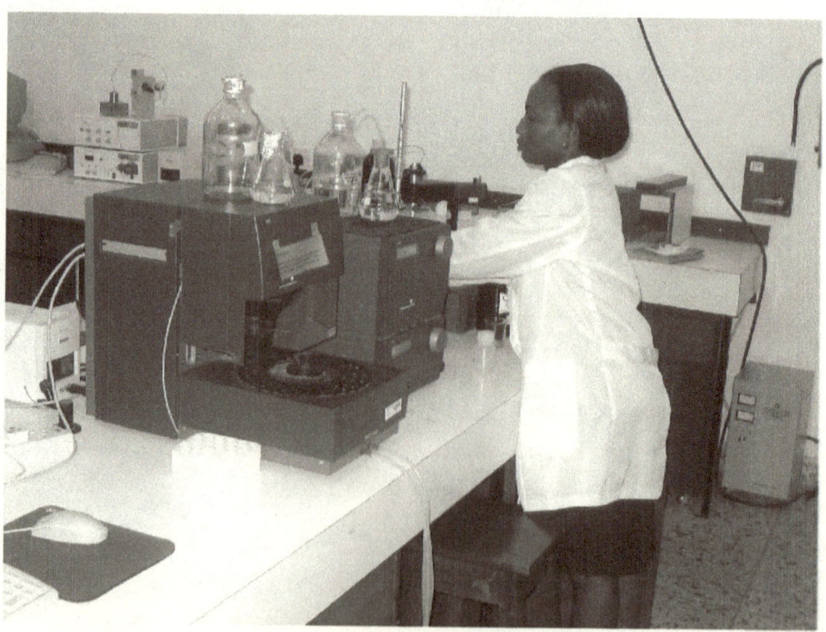

The Central Science Laboratory

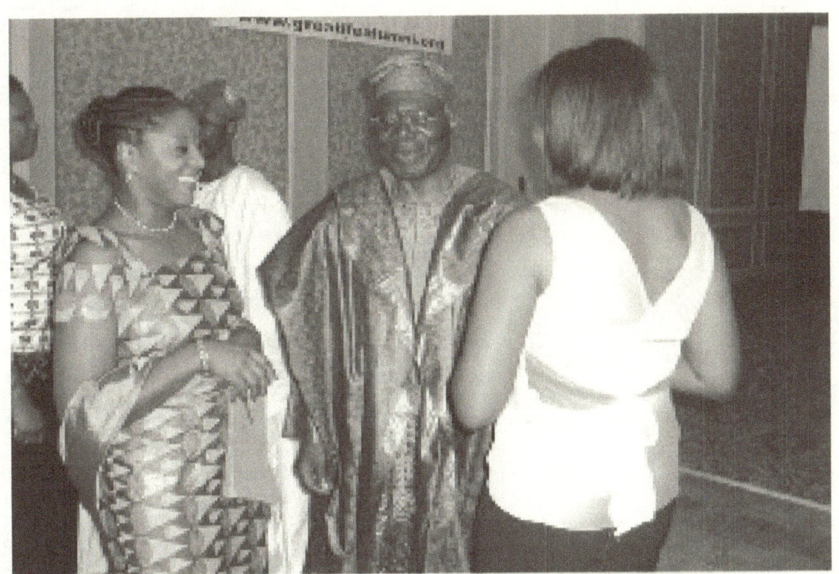

Houston Alumni Convention: on the left, the inaugural President, Yemi Koyejo, in the centre, Chief Ernest Shonekan, former Head of State

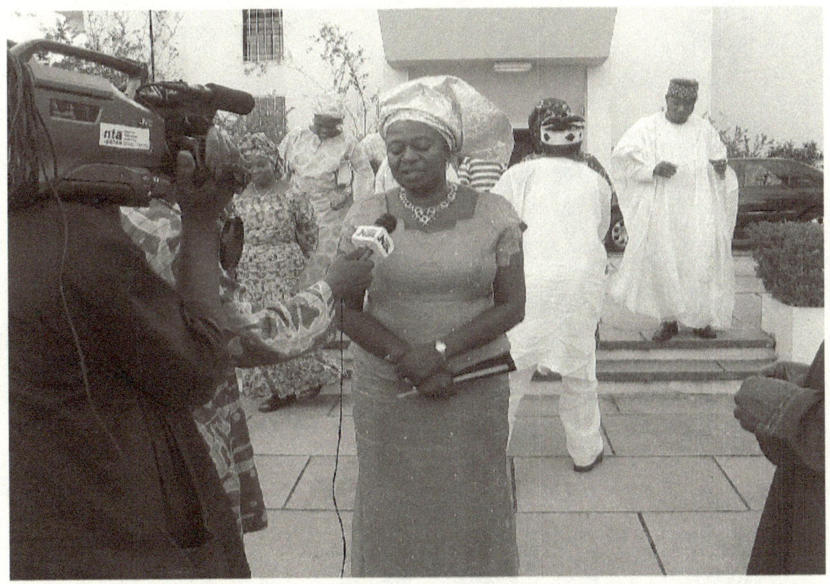

Erelu Olusola Obada, then Deputy Governor of Osun State, a true friend of the University, at a fund-raising programme at the VC's Lodge. In the background is Professor Wale Omole, my predecessor in office.

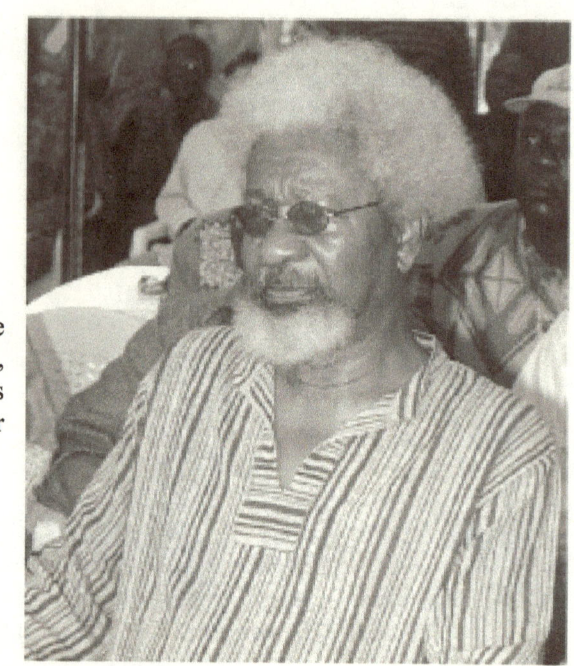

Nobel Laureate
Wole Soyinka,
He came back to Ife as
Emeritus Professor

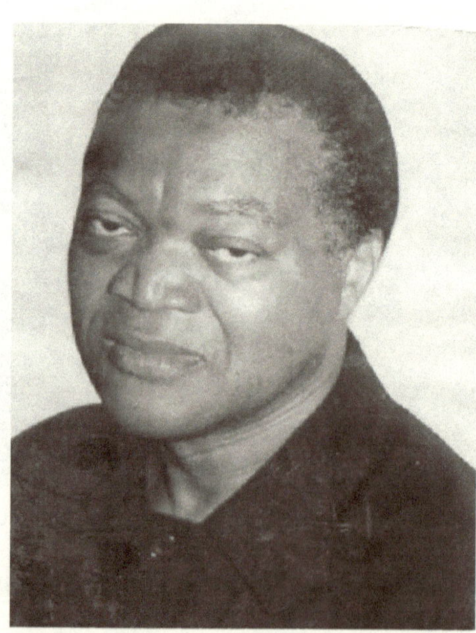

Professor
Olikoye Ransome-Kuti,
my mentor — a truly humane
man, an epitome
of hardwork, honesty
and honour

IX

Interlude—*Peace and Tranquility*

I spent a week in The Gambia, participating in my College's Annual General and Scientific Meeting. Actually, I spent more of that week relaxing than attending scientific sessions. At my request, I was booked into the *Bakadaji* Lodge, a relatively spartan but extremely tranquil place on Kololi beach. Towards the end of the conference, I gathered a few of my closest friends in the College and celebrated my "escape" from medical administration with wine, beer, and smoked chicken. I recommend The Gambia as the best place in West Africa to have a holiday.

As I relaxed in a beach chair, gazing at the ocean, I couldn't but look back in a reflective audit as to how my life had been shaped.

I was born in London on 4 April 1946, and was brought up by my maternal grandmother there until I was sent to the care of my paternal grandfather and uncle in Nigeria in December 1950.

My grandfather, Chief Olanimgbe Makanjuola, and my uncle, Richard Makanjuola, who later became the Oba (King) of Imesi-Ile, truly loved me and treated me as a very special but fragile child. Uncle Richard regarded me as his son. Our residences in the UK and in Ile-Ife are actually down to both of them. When my grandfather learnt I was taking up a job in Ile-Ife, he agreed to leave me a piece of land there. After his death, my uncle inherited most of his property, but, in accordance with his wishes, Uncle Richard transferred the piece of land to me. Dorothy and I started building on it in 1987 and I stayed in it for the first time in July 2011! It still doesn't have much furniture. That period with my grandfather and uncle in Ekotedo, Ibadan was a time of great privilege. Nothing was too good for me. It was believed that I would have difficulty with the local food, so my meals were delivered each day from the catering rest house.

When my father, Dr. Olatunde Makanjuola, returned to Nigeria in 1954, I re-joined the family. My biological mother is English. My father married a beautiful lady, Bamidele Familusi from his home town, Imesi-Ile. In spite of being a stepson, I was a loved member of the family. I have three sisters, Dele, Yombo and Kunbi, and a brother, Goke, who died. It was a happy, loving family. Initially, we lived in Ibadan, where I continued attending the University College, Ibadan Staff School. We moved to Lagos in 1955 and there I attended first St. Saviour's School and later the Corona Society School. In 1956 I went back to England and spent the next three years at the Yately Manor Preparatory School. I passed my entrance examination to Taunton Public School with high marks, but did not take up the admission. My father had come to Wales in 1958 to do a chest physicians' course and I went back to Nigeria with him in September 1959.

I entered King's College, Lagos in October 1959 and was thrown out of that school in December 1962 for an episode of vandalism. I should actually have been expelled, but the Principal, the famous P.H. Davis, merely withdrew the offer of a place in the Higher School Certificate class, because he felt I had been influenced by some older boys in my class. I was relatively naïve in those days and easily influenced by the others, who were two or more years older than I was at the time. The punishment was somewhat fortuitous, because I ended up entering university a year earlier than I should have done. My father and my Uncle Richard were extremely angry with me for being thrown out of school, but Uncle Richard got me into the Higher School Certificate class at Ibadan Grammar School. That was where I met the famous Canon Alayande, who was Principal of that school for so many years, and admired all over Western Nigeria for his headship of that institution. I came to respect him greatly. He was stern, indeed harsh, and with a somewhat precarious command of the English language, but all its graduates admitted that he ran the school very well and acknowledged the role Ibadan Grammar School had played in their development. On one occasion when he was a guest at a public lecture that I delivered I was able to publicly acknowledge his role in helping me. I stated that when I had been condemned, as it were, he had taken me on in spite of my bad reputation.

I only spent six months in that school, however. I took the concessional entrance examination to the University of Ibadan, passed and entered University in October 1963. Here I was lucky once more. When the results of the examination came out, my name was not on the Pass list. I knew I had done well, and my uncle went to see a friend, Mr. Fatodu, in the Registry of the University. Mr. Fatodu found that my main paper had not been marked because the examiner could not read my handwriting, and persuaded the examiner to mark it. I passed. Incidentally, my handwriting has always been a problem. The advent of the computer has solved that problem in recent years; I now type everything.

I spent seven happy years in the University of Ibadan. It was a six-year programme, but after my second MB examination, I was invited to take a year off to do a BSc in Physiological Sciences along with two others. As I just mentioned, I had a great time in the University. I worked hard, but I also played hard. I had a great social life, with, I am sorry to say (actually, I am not sorry at all!) rather great excesses, especially of alcohol. I drank copious quantities of beer, but when, as was so often the case, there was a paucity of funds, then we would go to Abadina (the junior staff quarters area) and buy *ogogoro* (illicit gin). It cost three shillings a bottle, and we would test it for strength by seeing how long it burned. We used to add various flavours to the raw spirit and tell the ladies it was Spanish Brandy!

I met my wife Dorothy in the University. I had known her since she came in in 1966, and we started going out in 1969, while we were doing our postings in psychiatry in Aro Hospital. We married on the 29 April 1972. People said our relationship would not last, but it has lasted 39 years and counting! In spite of my somewhat Bacchanalian lifestyle in University, I did very well academically. I was awarded three departmental prizes and five faculty prizes, including the Psychiatry prize, which influenced my decision to specialise in psychiatry. I was generally regarded as the best in my year.

After graduation, I worked as a house officer in the University College Hospital, Ibadan. As a reward for becoming a doctor, my grandfather bought me a red MG Midget, which was my pride and joy. I got into all sorts of escapades in it. My excesses continued. Like all young people, I took every opportunity to paint the town red. I remember one occasion when I drove from the Bristol Hotel on Lagos Island to the Caban Bamboo on the Ikorodu Road at about 1am on the wrong side of the road all the way. One of my passengers, a chap called Skido Martins was screaming in terror all the way. When we arrived at the night club, he staggered out mumbling "Thanks for nothing". They say God looks after young people. He certainly looked after me.

I was in two minds as to whether I should specialise in Obstetrics and Gynaecology or Psychiatry, both of which I had excelled in, winning the departmental prize in the first and the gold medal in the latter. Probably under the influence of Professor Thomas Adeoye Lambo, the famous psychiatrist, I eventually chose his discipline.

After ten months as a Senior House Officer in the University College Hospital, Ibadan, I travelled to Scotland and took up a job as Registrar at Rosslynlee Hospital, south of Edinburgh. This is where I gained most of my clinical training under Dr. Idwal Evans. At the end of one year, I was posted to the Medical Research Council Brain Metabolism Unit in the Royal Edinburgh

Hospital. We spent two afternoons each week on the training programme of the Department of Psychological Medicine of the University of Edinburgh, which was based at the Royal Edinburgh Hospital. The course comprised training for the Membership of the Royal College of Psychiatrists as well as the opportunity to do an MPhil degree. I took up that opportunity, so that I passed my Membership examination at the end of 1974 and was awarded my MPhil in October 1975. My research for the MPhil was in psychopharmacology, specifically on the behavioural effects of manipulation of monoamine transmitter pathways in rats, a project I did under the supervision of Professor George Ashcroft. George had a tremendous influence on my choice of academic career. He was a truly great man, kind and enthusiastic. He died in 2010. After the MPhil, I proceeded on to a PhD programme in the same field supervised by the late Dr. T.B.B. Crawford. Dr. Crawford and Professor Ashcroft were part of the group that demonstrated altered activity of brain serotonin systems in Affective Disorders. I obtained my PhD in October 1978. By then, Dorothy had also obtained the Fellowship of the Royal College of Radiologists.

Our time in Scotland was among the happiest of our lives. Our two children, Roger and Tony, were both born there. We were all extremely happy, and the boys had a fantastic upbringing. Edinburgh is a beautiful city and the surrounding area is also beautiful. Holyrood Park, in the middle of the city, has a mountain in its middle (actually, it is a high hill) called Arthur's Seat. There were other hills to the South and East. We used to climb them regularly. When the snows came in the winter, there was sledging, snowball fights and snowmen. Our children attended state nurseries and then state schools, but these were of very high standard.

We returned to Nigeria in October 1978 to take up lectureships in the University of Ife. That was the beginning of the love affair with Ife that has lasted for the rest of my life. As has been repeatedly, and perhaps monotonously, stated in other parts of this book, the Ife Campus is a true delight. It is a great place to bring up children. Our forays into the countryside that had been so much a part of our lives in Scotland were translated into equally enjoyable and educative forays into the various parts of the enormous Ife campus. The boys attended the University Staff School, which, under Mrs. Olugunna and then Mrs. Madeline Hollist, was extremely well run during their time there. Moremi High School opened in the late 1970s, and the boys transferred there when they were eleven. The further history of that school will come up subsequently; when our children were there, it was an excellent institution.

We were both actively teaching in the medical school, then called the Faculty of Health Sciences. The Faculty had been established by Professor T. Adesanya Ige Grillo virtually single-handed, and with a novel philosophy of providing medical education in the context of a comprehensive health care system encompassing the three levels of health care—Primary, Secondary and Tertiary (Specialist). Thus the associated teaching hospital complex took over health facilities as far as Imesi-Ile and, at least initially, Ondo. When we arrived, the "Complex" included two hospitals each in Ilesa and Ile-Ife as well as three health centres, in Ilesa, Ile-Ife and Imesi-Ile. It gradually retracted in the face of economic and political realities so that by the 1980s it was left with two major hospitals in Ilesa and Ile-Ife, a dental hospital on the University Campus and three health centres. A second innovation was that all the students of health sciences—medical, dental, nursing and physiotherapy—did a common four-year BSc Health Sciences programme before diverging into the clinical training in their various fields. The BSc programme ceased in the late 1980s, much to my regret, and the Faculty reverted to the traditional five-year programme of pre-clinical and clinical training after the one-year programme in the sciences. Professor Grillo was still there in 1978 when we arrived, but he was no longer the Dean. With the arrival of Professor Ojetunji Aboyade as Vice-Chancellor in 1975, a system of elections of Deans had been introduced. Professor Grillo lost the election to Professor M.A. Bankole, a paediatric surgeon. He took it badly and was still fuming when we arrived several months after the election.

A psychiatric unit had just been established at the Wesley Guild Hospital, Ilesa when we arrived, and I was posted there as its first consultant. I worked there for the rest of my career. Working with junior doctors and some dedicated nursing staff, the Unit developed into a very active mental health service. I believe we developed a great reputation as a source of help for this group of illnesses that was also the source of so much stigma. There were some particularly dedicated psychiatric nurses working with me, including G.O. Adeniji, M.A. Dada and Mrs. Awowoyin, who was nicknamed "Alhaja", in spite of the fact that she was a committed Christian; one day I will find out why. I had to travel to Ilesa up to four times weekly, but I did not mind that. I had been involved in the development of the unit, and I came to have a sense of belonging there. There was a great sense of camaraderie among all of us working there. I believe our clients also came to have faith in us.

My research focus in Edinburgh was psychopharmacology. I wanted to continue with this in Ife, but my productivity in this field was limited because of a lack of the required facilities. I concentrated on clinical research, particularly in the area of bipolar disorder, where I did make some impact. My interest in psychopharmacology also led me to develop an interest in traditional medicine. I carried out some studies on the efficacy of traditional medicine and discovered that Yoruba traditional healers were effective in the management of psychotic disorders and mania. However, I also discovered that these healers keep their patients in their establishments for far too long, often for months after I assessed them as clinically recovered. This was often because they had not paid their "hospital" bills, which might run into tens of thousands of naira. The project I enjoyed most was the one in which I had to identify the various agents that traditional healers use, which included plants, minerals, oils, and various exotic animals. I collected and identified over one hundred and sixty plants that these healers use. Probably the most significant one is *Rauwolfia vomitoria*, known by the Yoruba as *Asofeyeje* as well as a variety of other names signifying its properties, such as *elegbon were* ("the older brother of madness") and *apawere* ("the killer of madness"). I had a great time collecting the specimens. This was a project, i.e., work, that allowed me to indulge one of my favourite pastimes—walking. I spent many happy hours tramping through the bush, accompanied by different traditional healers, collecting these specimens. A botanist, Dr. Jayeola, worked with me on identifying them. After a while, I became quite proficient at identifying them myself, using the reference books that are employed for that purpose as well as reference herbarium specimens.

Both Dorothy and I made fairly rapid progress up the academic hierarchy. I experienced some antagonism within my department, and I had to petition for each of my promotions to senior lecturer, Reader and Professor. That is another great thing about Ife—it is an institution where you will always get justice. Dorothy became a professor in 1985 and I achieved that status in 1984.

Our joy in the Ife campus continued unabated. We took up fishing; the delights of fishing in Ife will be attended to in great detail later. Both Roger and Tony became very proficient anglers. We used to catch large quantities of fish most Saturdays. On some occasions when the fish were biting vigorously, the fish would be reeled in so fast that I would stop and sit or stand between them, unhooking the tilapia as they hauled them in. We also took up cricket. After a youth corper introduced the game to Moremi High School, a group of us in the Staff Club decided to form a team to play against the school team. That was the beginning of a really enjoyable period. The Ife Cricket Club played teams from all over Western Nigeria. We enjoyed the games and enjoyed the après games even more—a good lunch, good drinks and great camaraderie. We used to thrash a team from Ibadan captained by Kolade Mosuro regularly. Even more importantly, most of the close friendships that I have were established through this club.

This is my background, the upbringing that has influenced the rest of my life, including my professional and personal values, which I took into my role as an administrator.

Two days after my return from The Gambia , I was on a plane to London. We have a small flat there, which I purchased in 1988 from the proceeds of the sale of a larger residence that my grandfather had left me in his will. My plan was to work in the UK as a psychiatrist, and earn some real money. I was actually less well off financially at the end of my term as CMD than before I took up the appointment. I had already enquired from the General Medical Council (GMC) as to my eligibility for registration and for employment as a consultant and received the reassuring reply that I was eligible to be placed on the specialist register, having worked as a consultant in 1988 when I took a sabbatical in Aberdeen. When I presented myself to the Council after my arrival, I found that things were not quite that simple. I was informed that I was indeed eligible for placement on the Specialist Register in Psychiatry, but could only be placed on that Register if I was licensed to practice. I was eligible for Limited Registration, but would have to pass an English test and be appointed first as a junior doctor. Once I was granted Limited Registration, I would automatically be eligible for the Specialist Register, and once I was on that Register, I would automatically be eligible for full registration! The wheels of bureaucracy are very much in evidence, even in the UK.

I was in trouble. I could either go the route of an English test and a junior doctor's position or I would have to return home. I decided to stay. I found the centre that was going to organise the English test as soon as I could and booked for it. The test is called the International English Language Test System (IELTS) and has to be taken by most foreign professionals from outside the European Union who wish to work in the UK. When I phoned to book the examination I was asked whether I was an examiner! As those who have met me know, my English is fairly good. I travelled up to Colchester and took the examination. The examiner gave me my result on the spot, and armed with it, I started applying for jobs as a locum Senior House Officer. I did one week in Runwell Hospital and then three weeks in Ford, both in Essex. In the first hospital, I found that two of the junior doctors were individuals whom I had taught in Ife, and that they occupied positions slightly more senior than mine! I must say that we got on well, and they were very helpful. In the second hospital, when the consultant learnt that I had the Membership of the Royal College of Psychiatrists, and, following a few days during which he appraised my skills, he would happily leave me to look after the patients while he went off to his private practice or to play golf.

Towards the end of that month working as a junior doctor, I received a letter from the GMC stating that I was, after all, eligible for full registration as well as to be placed on the Specialist Register. While I had been trying to sort out my registration, a former teacher of mine had angrily informed the President of the Royal College of Psychiatrists of the situation. The latter had intervened with the President of the GMC, and the Council had reviewed the situation. Thus, if I had waited, I would not have had to go through the "embarrassment" of taking up a junior doctor's position. Actually, I was not embarrassed at all. My initial period as a Senior House Officer did provide me with valuable experience. I was able to familiarise myself with the psychiatric system in the country, especially with the newer treatments that were not yet available in Nigeria, and with the new mental health legislation. If I had gone straight into a consultant's position, I would have had difficulties. More importantly, I earned money during the one-month period. I was paid weekly, and in my second week, when I was on call for long periods, I earned over one thousand pounds!

Armed with my full registration as a psychiatrist, I spent the next eight months working as a consultant at Napsbury Hospital, London Colney. I was in charge of an acute psychiatric service, and also was involved in the rehabilitation into the community of two groups of chronically ill patients. It was very rewarding work. I truly felt I was making a difference to the lives of sick people, and I believe I was highly respected for my expertise as well as my commitment to patient care. Equally important, the pay was good. My father died towards the end of my sojourn in the UK. If I had not done that work in England, I would have been placed in the shameful position of not being able to pay for his funeral.

It was great being in England. I enjoyed the work. I had fine colleagues. In particular, there was Ian Fulton, a community psychiatric nurse. He had started his professional life as a lawyer, but had given this up to go into psychiatric nursing. He shared my commitment to the care of patients. His long experience in the system made his advice very valuable to me. We shared an interest in the countryside and also in countryside pubs, although my high regard for beer was somewhat greater than his.

There was only one time when I found the work stressful. A patient with drug and personality problems was referred by his Probation Officer because of an apparent worsening of his mental state. He had a previous conviction for causing grievous bodily harm. Ian had earlier informed me of his suspicion that the patient had committed a murder. I made the mistake of seeing him on my own. He was extremely disturbed and highly aroused. Throughout the interview, he threatened violence. I felt myself to be in serious danger. In the end, to my relief, he stormed out. I later learnt that there was an alarm button under my desk which I could have used to call for help, but, as they say, knowledge after the fact has no value. Unfortunately, the Probation Officer phoned me again later that day to state that the patient was a serious suicidal risk. I had to go to his house that evening to evaluate him. However, this time, I went with two policemen, who, when they were informed of the episode of grievous bodily harm, had armed themselves with "mace," a form of tear gas. I met his mother, a pleasant old lady, at the door, and subsequently interviewed the patient upstairs, with the police on stand-by on the stairs. This time, he was extremely pleasant. He told me of his frustration over his life. On enquiry, he admitted that his current placid state was because he had just smoked some "blow" (cannabis).

I was working in a rural area, and after work, I would go for long rambles in the countryside. I saw all sorts of birds. In the summer, there were lots of rabbits, and I saw a few foxes. At the weekend, I would travel back to London, to spend the period with Tony. Roger was then studying law at Warwick while Tony was doing a Masters' degree at Imperial College. Walks around London, beer, and a care-free life made life real good.

I went back to Nigeria in April for the College examinations as I was Chief Examiner of the Faculty of Psychiatry at that time. I visited France twice—boy, do they have good wine there!

I finally returned to Nigeria at the end of September 1998. My sisters and I had the unhappy task of burying our father. Fortunately, my sister Dele, the one next to me, had organised everything to perfection. There was a huge turnout of our friends and colleagues as well as those of my father. It all went very well, with much celebration. He was 79 years old. However, as much as all went well, I can never come to terms with this practice of dancing around with the coffin and even throwing it into the air and catching it. They also did this to Professor Grillo's corpse shortly afterwards. T. Adesanya Ige Grillo, my anatomy teacher and mentor, was a very straight-laced black "Englishman." As they were tossing him about on the way to the cemetery, I said to myself, "He will turn in his grave"! May the soul of my father, Dr. Olatunde Makanjuola, rest in perfect peace.

I returned to the University and resumed my duties as a teacher and consultant. I also got right back into the BFI, which had continued to record major successes. B-Zone, for which I was still Coordinator, and Osun State, continued to lead the way, with more and more health facilities being designated Baby Friendly, and more and more families adopting proper breast feeding practices.

During my interlude in the peaceful atmosphere of England, I had decided that I would run for the Vice-Chancellorship of the University whenever the position opened. I felt that I had a good chance based on my record in the hospital. The incumbent, Professor Wale Omole, was due to leave the post at the end of 1999, and by the time I got back to Ife, campaigning had already started. I did mention my intention to a few friends, but did not go out campaigning. However, I started preparing a document on the University, with an evaluation of its achievements and weaknesses and proposals for the future. In preparing this document, I consulted with key individuals concerning various aspects of its functions.

The post was advertised in April 1999. The system of appointments of Vice-Chancellors provides for a Search Party consisting of members of Council and Senate "to identify and nominate individuals who are not likely to apply for the post of their own volition, because they feel it is not proper to do so." For obvious reasons, it was generally considered that it was better to be "searched" than to apply. However, the system had been corrupted, with aspirants actively lobbying to be "searched." I decided to apply straightaway. The search party did approach me, and I informed the team that I had already applied. I printed my manifesto and also got it circulated on the University's intranet. That was my campaign. It was the habit of candidates to go from person to person campaigning, and even to visit members of staff in their homes. I did not approach a single person, although when members of staff approached me, I would speak with them for as long as they wished. My campaign was my manifesto. Since all of the other contestants were busy going from person to person, which the average Nigerian, whatever their status, seemed to expect, I must have come across as quite arrogant. The truth is that I believe persons seeking a position such as Vice-Chancellor of a university need to act in a dignified manner, and parading themselves from place to place, begging for support, is not consistent with that. More worrying is the fact that, in Nigeria, individuals seeking positions lobby heavily among those who may influence the appointment. Thus, several of the contestants made repeated visits to Abuja, looking for godfatherly influence. I did not go anywhere.

Apart from seeking human intervention, many candidates resorted to *juju*. There were charms and sacrifices everywhere. Late one night, a completely naked individual carrying a load on his head ran down a road in the Senior Staff Quarters, shouting, *A ayiwo, o* ("We do not look at this, o"). Those in the surrounding houses were scared, and stayed locked up in their homes. However, as he was proceeding, a young student returning from a religious service came across him and started shouting; "In the name of Jesus!" The apparition ran!

As had become the practice, the local branch of the Academic Staff Union of Universities (ASUU) organised a referendum. The law did not provide for an input into the appointment by any union, but the results of the referendum were normally sent to the Governing Council and there is no doubt that it did influence the decisions of that body. ASUU also organised an interactive session during which each candidate would address the members of the union and answer questions. We were requested to provide 1200 copies of a summary of our manifestos. I sent 1200 copies of my full 20-page manifesto. I was examining in Benin at the time of the interactive session, and travelled back to Ife on the day appointed for me. I thought the session went well. I did receive one or two hostile questions, including one from Dr. Idowu Awopetu who said that I had done my best to eliminate unionism in the hospital. To this I answered with the Churchillian quotation, "That is a terminological inexactitude." I wonder if he has yet found out the meaning of that term! I got the impression that most of the audience, particularly the young lecturers, were quite enthusiastic about me. One of the points I had made very strongly in my manifesto was that we should work to eliminate corruption. I made the point that corruption at all levels should be dealt with and that, *Thief na thief.* When I raised the issue during my initial address, one of the young lecturers shouted, *Thief na thief,* to loud and exultant acclaim. The referendum was organised the next day and I won by a landslide. I was later informed that the ASUU leadership was very unhappy about the outcome, as their favoured candidates had not received much support. Although the results of the referendum were announced, they were never released to the Press. The Senior Staff Association of Nigerian Universities (SSANU) also organised an interactive session and a referendum. I reluctantly participated in that and again, won the referendum by a clear margin.

My academic colleagues and the rest of the senior staff had expressed their preference for me in the Vice-Chancellorship race. The younger members of academic staff were particularly enthusiastic. It was now left to the Governing Council to make its decision. In accordance with the law, the interviews of applicants were to be conducted by a Joint Committee of Council and Senate, which would recommend a number of candidates to the Governing Council for its consideration. I thought my interview went very well, and was reasonably confident that I would be among those recommended for the final consideration of the Governing Council. I was flabbergasted when the news filtered out that I had been rated tenth out of twelve candidates. I believe many other members of the Community felt the same. Eventually, the Council recommended three individuals for the post to the Government. These were the two current Deputy Vice-Chancellors and a former Deputy VC who had worked with the outgoing VC. I mention this because there was some speculation that the tragic events that followed soon afterwards were in part influenced by this.

I was terribly disappointed. I wrote an open letter to the University Community thanking them for their support. At the end of the letter, I quoted Edmund Burke's assertion, "The only thing necessary for the triumph of evil is for good men (I added "and good women") to do nothing." I really should not have included that quotation; it reeked of bitterness. I left a few days later for a breastfeeding training course in London, in which I became completely engrossed. I was also in the midst of my family, and was soon able to get over my bitter disappointment. One week into the course, I phoned my friend, Olu "Oga" Arigbabu. His first words were, "The situation is very tense." He gave me the news of an invasion of the University Campus by a secret cult, and that some students had been killed. Four days later, I travelled to Oxford with the other members of the breastfeeding course. On arrival at the Radcliffe Infirmary in Oxford, as we were entering the building, a receptionist hailed us, asking for "Dr. Makanjuola." She said I was to phone a number in London urgently. The number was that of my flat in London, and my son, Tony's fiancée, Wanne, answered and informed me that the Minister of Education was trying to contact me. She gave me two numbers. One was that of Professor 'Tunde Adeniran, the Federal Minister of Education, the other was that of Dr. Lola Borishade, Special Adviser on Education to the President. I was able to call the Minister. He told me that I had been appointed Acting Vice-Chancellor and that I should return to Nigeria immediately to take up the post. I agreed without hesitation. I subsequently phoned some of my close friends in Ife, who all advised that I should take up the task. Thus, I had to cut short my course half way through, and book my early return to Nigeria. I flew back on the night of Sunday 18 July and drove immediately to Ile-Ife, arriving about 11pm.

X

Into the Fiery Furnace —
The Black Axe Murders

The full story of what happened in Ife on the night of 10 July 1999 is not totally clear. However, the version that follows is based on various accounts and the proceedings of the Judicial Commission of Enquiry that investigated the incident and my interpretations.

The beginnings of the secret cult phenomenon in Nigeria are unfairly traced back to the Pyrates Confraternity, which was established in the 1950s by 'Wole Soyinka and some other students in the University College, Ibadan, (now University of Ibadan [UI]). I believe that the Pyrates Confraternity was not a secret cult. I was a student at UI in the 1960s, and there was no secret about either their membership or their activities. I knew many of their members, and their activities were quite open and quite innocuous, though rather boisterous. It is possible that their culture subsequently evolved in the direction of what we now call "cultism;" if so, then this occurred well after my own time as a university student.

The original Pyrates Confraternity changed its name to the National Association of Seadogs some years ago, and this Association has as its members "Pyrates" from the earlier days.

That Association is a registered society. There is one secret cult called "The Pirates", but it appears to have no connection with the original Pyrates Confraternity.

During the 1970s, a substantial number of truly secret cults emerged, and began to expand, both in their membership and their geographical spread. These societies are secret cults; their activities and their membership are secret. They also have secret rituals. Many of their activities are anti-social; members carry a variety of weapons, and maimings and killings are common— both of cult members and innocent victims who incur their wrath. However, membership does incur some "benefits" such as protection, a sense of belonging, and even patronage. The system can be likened to the Street Gang phenomenon of many industrialised nations, with its activities and rituals coloured by local cultural influences. Among the most prominent secret cults are the Black Axe, the *Buccaneers*, and the *Eiye* Confraternity. The secret cult scourge affects most universities and polytechnics in Nigeria, but the problem is greater in the south. A worrying development in recent years is the expansion of some cults even into secondary schools. Secret cult membership is for life. It continues after the individual leaves university, and it is said that some of these societies wield great influence within the Nigerian political system.

In Ife, the secret cult problem became a serious menace from the 1980s. There had been episodes of individuals being accused of "cultism", with varying degrees of evidence. In 1995, there was a major clash between members of two secret cults, the Black Axe and the Mafites in the vicinity of the Religious Centre, arising out of a dispute over a girl. Some of the combatants were injured and had to be taken to hospital. Clearly, this was a serious problem for the university. Only a small minority of students were involved, but they were wreaking havoc. There were claims in the past that some Student Union leaders were cult members. Whether this is true or not, in the period preeceding 10 July 1999, the student leadership was actively engaged in combating secret cults in the University. Even though the Student Union had been proscribed at this particular period because of their violent protests, they still wielded de facto leadership and enjoyed recognition among the students.

On Saturday, 7 March 1999, a group of Black Axe members held a meeting in Ife town. After the meeting, they drove back to the campus. On the main road, Road 1, leading into the campus, they were overtaken by some students in another car. For whatever reason, they were enraged and gave chase to the students. The students, seeing them in pursuit, raced hastily to the car park outside Angola Hall and ran into the adjacent Awolowo Hall for safety. The Students' Union, which had also received information that secret cult members were gathering in a house in the senior staff quarters, mobilised in response to the incident. Led by George Iwilade, the Secretary-General, a group of them drove to the house, officially occupied by Mr. F.M. Mekoma, and forced their way into the boys' quarters. They found nine individuals inside, eight of them students of the University, with a submachine gun, a locally manufactured gun, an axe, a bayonet and the black clothing and regalia of the Black Axe cult. The University authorities were informed, and the members of the secret cult were handed over to the Police. They were held in police custody and taken to the Chief Magistrate's Court where two weeks later they were granted bail.

The case was heard on 31 March, and to the utmost amazement of everyone, the Chief Magistrate discharged and acquitted the arrested individuals. The students who had apprehended the cult members were not called as witnesses. The investigating police officer, Corporal Femi Adewoye, claimed that the witnesses could not be located and actually stated in Court, "I tried to contact the complainants in this case, all to no avail. To date, there is no complainant in the case. Since all the accused persons denied the allegations against them and there is no complainant, there is no way the allegations can be proved." This was the submission of the prosecuting police officer! Usually, in such cases, witness' summons were served through the University Administration but this did not happen. The trial was concluded in two court appearances in eight days.

The Chief Magistrate also ordered that the submachine gun be sent to the police armourer and the other exhibits be destroyed, thus eliminating all the evidence, and making it impossible to re-open the case. The Judicial Enquiry recommended that the Magistrate be reported to the Judicial Commission for appropriate disciplinary action. Nothing came of this, as nothing came of all the other recommendations of that Panel.

After the arrests of the cult members, the University, under pressure from the students, issued a release suspending them without serving them with letters of suspension. Shortly afterwards, the University was closed as a result of a student crisis. When it re-opened three months later, the cult members returned to the campus and were seen attending lectures. The students raised an alarm once more. In response to this, the University issued a release on 2 July re-affirming the suspensions of the cult members. The letters of suspension were dated 8 July and it is doubtful whether those affected actually received them before the tragic events two days later. Even then, one of the students, Bruno Arinze, was left out. I eventually suspended him on 23 July.

The cult involved in the episode of 7 March was the Black Axe. Four major reasons have been advanced as to the genesis leading to the mayhem on 10 July. One, to which I subscribe, was that the Black Axe was avenging the humiliating treatment of its members by the Student Union leaders in March. A second, more complex and much less credible theory was that the attacks were motivated by enmity towards the VC, even though the enemies were not identified. According to this theory, the instigators of the attack saw the VC as trying to put a favoured deputy in place as his successor. The attacks would have put the University into chaos and discredited the incumbent VC. This certainly did happen, but I find it difficult to give credibility to such a tangled web of intrigue.

A third theory, which the students advanced quite forcibly, was that the VC had paid the secret cult members to prosecute the attack, in the course of which they were to eliminate the student leaders who were giving his administration so much trouble.

I do not find this theory credible at all. Finally, a faction of the students' leadership claimed that the attacks were organised by a rival faction within the Students' Union with which they were at loggerheads. This made absolutely no sense, because Lanre Adeleke, whose faction was the one accused of instigating the attacks, was in the same camp as George Iwilade, the Secretary-General, who was one of those killed.

On the night of 9 July 1999, the *Kegites*, members of the Palm Wine Drinkers' Club, held a "gyration" (party) in the cafeteria of Awolowo Hall. The party was in full swing, when, at around 3.30am (now 10 July), a group of masked individuals, wearing black clothing, drove through the main gate and proceeded to the car park next to the Tennis Courts in the Sports Centre. They disembarked there and went on foot along a bush path to Awolowo Hall, where they violently interrupted the gyration, firing guns and also wielding axes and cutlasses. The group was probably all young men, although there is a persistent story of at least one woman among them. Some of the partygoers were shot, though none of them was killed. The partygoers ran for their lives, a few actually throwing themselves through glass doors. A group of the gunmen chased the partygoers as far as Mozambique Hall. Other groups proceeded to the rooms. They first entered Room 184, where they shot and killed Efe Ekede, a Part II Psychology student. In Room 230, they shot Charles Ita, a Part II Law student. A group of the attackers then shot Yemi Ajiteru, a Part II Religious Studies student, through the head in the corridor outside the Kegites' headquarters. In Room 273, they found George Iwilade (Afrika), the Secretary-General of the Students' Union and a Law student, and shot him through the head, along with another occupant, Tunde Oke, a Part 1 student of Philosophy, who was shot in the abdomen. When the attackers got to Room 271, the room allocated to the suspended Students' Union President, Lanre Adeleke (Legacy), they found that he had escaped. Legacy was in his room when he heard the first gun shots. He hurriedly went to his door, looked out, and saw two of the attackers on the next floor, firing shots. He ran back into his room and broke through the partition of the kitchenette into the next room's kitchenette. He heard them shouting, "Legacy, come out!" and escaped into the next room. During the course of the incident, the attackers also shouted the names of "Afrika", George Iwilade, and "Dexter", the Chief of the Kegites, demanding that they come out. The band of thugs proceeded to Fajuyi Hall on foot, where they shot and killed one more student. That individual, Eviano Ekelemo, a medical student, was certainly not a student activist, but they shot him anyway. The murderers left Fajuyi Hall on foot and went through the bush path behind the Hall back to their vehicles. They drove to the Students' Union building, which they ransacked. They returned to their vehicles and drove out of the University through the main gate. The security staff, having heard gunfire, fled for their lives. Thus the exit of the marauding thugs was unchallenged.

The students with gunshot wounds were taken to the Health Centre and from there to the Teaching Hospital. Tunde Oke was still alive but died on the operating table. Four others, George Iwilade, Yemi Ajiteru, Efe Ekede and Eviano Ekelemu, were brought in dead. Eviano Ekelemu bled to death from gunshot wounds to the groin and thigh. The other three died from gunshot wounds to the head. In each case, the weapons used were shotguns, fired at close range. Charles Ita and five others who were shot in the Awolowo Hall cafeteria, survived. Twenty-five others received minor injuries, which were sustained during the stampede out of the Awolowo Hall cafeteria and later on during the attack.

In the aftermath of the attack, the whole university was enveloped in fear and there was chaos in the halls of residence. However, within a short time, the President of the Students' Union, Lanre Adeleke, was able to restore order and mobilise his colleagues. The students went to the town searching for the perpetrators in locations where cult members were thought to be living. They "arrested" three indivduals and brought them back to Awolowo Hall. These were Aisekhaghe Aikhile, a Part I student of Agricultural Economics, Emeka Ojuagu, and Frank Idahosa (Efosa). Efosa and Ojuagu were arrested in a public transport vehicle that was about to leave Ife. The students exhibited black clothing, two berets and two T-shirts, that had been found in Ojuagu's bag, which was claimed to be the Black Axe uniform. Efosa was a known member of the Black Axe. He had been expelled from the University of Benin and was later admitted for a diploma programme in Local Government Studies in Ife. The three of them were savagely beaten and tortured in the Awolowo Hall "Coffee Room", the traditional venue for such events. The inverted commas have been employed because coffee had not been known to be served there for many years. Efosa and Oguagu are said to have confessed to participating in the attacks during their "interrogation", and Efosa is said to have gone further to state that the attack was organised to avenge the humiliating treatment of the Black Axe members who had been arrested in Mr. Mekoma's house on 7 March. At a hastily arranged student congress later that morning, he made a further statement that the attack was organised on the orders of Professor Wale Omole, the VC. It is difficult to give credibility to this latter statement which was made after extremely brutal torture.

In the course of the interrogation, Aisekhaghe Aikhile died, and his body was taken to the hospital mortuary. There was a subsequent claim by some of the students that Aisekhaghe Ikhile was actually shot dead in error by his own comrades during the attack. However, the autopsy showed that Aisekhaghe Ikhile had been brutally beaten, and that his death was as a result of a broken neck. He was not shot. Efosa and Ojuagu were handed over to the Police, with Ojuagu being admitted to the Teaching Hospital as a result of his injuries. The interrogations also yielded the information that 22 Black Axe members were involved, six from the University, four from the University of Lagos, four from the University of Ibadan, and eight from the University of Calabar. There was also a separate claim that more students from the University of Benin were also involved.

Another young man, Olufemi Samuel, not a student, but alleged to be a member of the *Eiye* Confraternity, was picked up in the town a few days after the attacks and also subjected to brutal interrogation. His body was taken to the mortuary by student leaders on 14 July. The autopsy showed that he had died as a result of severe head injuries.

The VC, Professor Wale Omole, had been out of the country on 10 July 1999, the day of the attack and in his absence, the Deputy VC (Academic), Professor A.E. Akingbohungbe, was in charge. Professor Femi Ajibola, the Deputy VC (Administration), was the first member of the Administration to be alerted about the incident at around 5.30am. Professor Ajibola informed Professor Akingbohungbe and then linked up with the Director of Corporate Affairs, Mr. Femi Idowu, and they both proceeded to the Police Headquarters in More, Ile-Ife to report the incident. On the way, they met the Welfare Officer of the Students' Union, who gave them more information about the incident. They all proceeded to the Police Area Command where they reported the attacks.

The principal officers of the University and a few of the senior academic staff held a meeting in the afternoon to review the situation. The principal officers were advised not to go to the halls of residence because of the possibility of attack by aggrieved students. At the end of the meeting, a press release was issued on the incident and a delegation went to the hospital to see to the welfare of the students who had been taken there. Professor Ajibola travelled to Osogbo that evening to meet with the Commissioner of Police. The Commissioner immediately dispatched a contingent of mobile policemen to the campus. They arrived later that evening. It was agreed that the Commissioner should come to the University the following morning, reporting at the VC's Lodge, and that he and the university principal officers would then proceed to the halls of residence to meet with the students and inspect the scene of the murders. The principal officers waited in vain for him the next day. Rather than reporting at the VC's Lodge, the Commissioner went straight to the halls of residence and met with the students. Later that morning, the Commissioner showed up at the VC's Lodge and stated that he had gone to the University Staff Club at the appointed hour, and finding no one there, had proceeded to the halls.

The students held a congress at around 8 o'clock that morning. Professor Ajibola had been invited to address the congress, but declined, presumably because of fears for his own safety. During the congress, Efosa made his statement concerning the involvement of the VC. Immediately afterwards, rampaging groups of students proceeded to the senior staff quarters. They first attacked the residence of Professor Ajibola and then that of Professor Akingbohungbe. By the time they arrived, both had vacated their residences, along with their families, based on a security report about the resolution of the Congress. The students damaged their residential buildings, but mainly externally. Ostensibly in the search for the attackers, they also entered the Conference Centre, where they went from room to room, claiming to be searching for the murderers and harassing the residents in the process. They are alleged to have ransacked the bar and drunk or removed substantial quantities of alcohol. They also went to the VC's Lodge, but could not get in. As a result of the attacks, both Deputy VCs had to go into hiding with their families, as did the Dean of Student Affairs, Professor D.O. Kolawole. It was reported that these officers had been declared "wanted persons" by the students during the congress. There was at least one report that a "death sentence" had been passed on the VC by the Students' Union. This was probably just a rumour, but it does illustrate the depth of the chaos the university had been plunged into.

At some point on the day of the murders, a group of students went to Osogbo where they forcibly removed Efosa from police custody. They took him to Lagos for a press conference the following day and returned him to the Police afterwards.

There was a mass exodus of students from the campus in the aftermath of the murders. During that exodus, Seyi Ojewale, a Part IV Economics student, died in a road traffic accident.

The campus was in a state of anarchy, with both staff and students in fear, not just of attack by secret cult members, but also of attacks from students.

The VC returned from his trip to the campus the night after the tragedy. The members of the University Administration did not go to the halls for fear of attacks by students, and this must have further exacerbated the hostility towards the Administration and the suspicions which the students had about them. The Registrar, Mrs. Bola Iluyomade, pleaded that they should go and talk with the students, but she was overruled. This is particularly noteworthy, since, some months before, Mrs. Iluyomade had been held hostage by the students and badly treated. A brave woman, indeed. Efforts to initiate interactions between the students and the University Administration by the Academic Staff Union of Universities (ASUU) and by a Committee of Elders that had been set up by the Administration to liaise with the students both failed. One invitation to a meeting on 17 July was rejected by the students who demanded that the letter should be addressed officially to the "President of the Students' Union." Technically, this could not be done since the Administration had suspended the Students' Union and its executive some months earlier. The VC's wife, Sade Omole, was kidnapped by students from a church service on the campus in the afternoon of Wednesday, 14 July and held for two hours before she was released. She was not physically harmed, but one can only imagine the terror she endured in the hands of the students, who were convinced her husband was behind the murders.

Soon after his arrival, the VC was summoned to Abuja to give a report of the incident the day after he returned to campus. On 14 July, his suspension was announced by the Government. It was against this background that I was tracked to the UK and summoned to return immediately and assume duty as the acting VC of the University.

When I arrived on the campus on 18 July, I promised the students and the rest of the university community, that the university would do everything in its power to bring the perpetrators to justice. I took this undertaking extremely seriously. The first step was to visit the Commissioner of Police, Mr. J.C. Nwoye, in Osogbo. I raised the issue of the nine individuals who had been arrested in March and discharged by the Chief Magistrate. He promised that a vigorous and thorough investigation was in progress on the matter. He then expressed concern that the University authorities had not officially reported the murders to the Police despite repeated requests. On my return to the University, I wrote the required letter, once more indicating our strong fears concerning a connection between the March episode and the murders, and requesting that the nine individuals involved be re-arrested.

A total of 12 individuals were arrested and charged to court over the three weeks following the murders, including Efosa and Ojuagu. Only one of those involved in the March episode was among those arrested. The other eight could not be located. Two of them had obtained their transcripts and resumed their studies in France. The students brought information on the whereabouts of a major suspect, Babatunde Kazeem (Kato), and we provided a vehicle so that the Police could go with the students to the address in Lagos and arrest him. Kato was a former student who had been "advised to withdraw" from the University as a result of academic failure. He had been apprehended by the Students' Union in August 1997 when he admitted to being a secret cult member. He was subsequently handed over to the Security Department, but there is no record of what happened after that. We also provided the Police with information on three other individuals, "Innocent", "Yuletide" and "Ogbume." Sadly, nothing came of this, even though we provided Ogbume's address in Victoria Garden City, Lagos. The arrested persons were charged to the Ile-Ife Magistrate's court for the murders.

After the first hearing of the charges in the Magistrate's Court, there was a near-riot in the court premises, as irate students beat up the lawyer representing Efosa. As a result of this, the case was transferred to the Magistrate's Court in Osogbo. I attended most of the subsequent hearings at the Magistrate's Court and the High Court, along with the University's legal officer. The students also attended in large numbers, and there was increasing concern over the security of the accused persons, their counsel, and even the court officials during the hearings. On one occasion, I had to give an undertaking to the Chief Magistrate over the behaviour of our students.

Eventually, only three of the arrested individuals, Efosa, Kato, and Ojuagu, were arraigned before the Osogbo High Court on the charge of conspiring to kill and the murders of the five students. The others were charged in the Magistrate's Court for belonging to an illegal organisation. That latter case gradually petered out and the accused persons were eventually discharged. It is likely that several of those involved in the latter case were actually innocent. One had renounced his secret cult membership before 10 July and three others had convincing alibis.

The students continually complained about the investigation and prosecution of the 10 July murders. I was also not happy and nor was our legal unit. We were also concerned about the delay in setting up the promised Judicial Commission. I travelled to Abuja and met with the Minister of Justice. I expressed the concern of the University and its students over the delay. He initially indicated that the Government was considering setting up an administrative rather than a judicial panel. I stressed the fact that the students had expressed trust in his promise of a Judicial Commission and that only a Judicial Commission would satisfy the nation. He agreed to put the case for a Judicial Commission to the Head of State.

The Judicial Commission of Enquiry was eventually inaugurated in Abuja on 18 October, but did not start work until 24 November, and eventually arrived in the University on Sunday, 28 November. The Chairman was Justice Okoi Itam. There were six other members, including Professor Jadesola Akande, an experienced and highly respected academic and university administrator, and Ray Ekpu, the journalist. Ms. Turi Akerele was later deployed as legal counsel to the Commission. A flamboyant but highly capable alumnus, Adeyinka Olumide-Fusika, led a team representing the students. I was extremely impressed by this lawyer's commitment to obtaining justice for the murdered students, though he was probably biased in favour of one student faction. Chief Akin Olujimi, the University's legal adviser, represented the University. There was also legal representation on behalf of Professor Wale Omole and the family of George Iwilade.

I attended the sittings that took place in the Oduduwa Hall amphitheatre over a one-month period. Fifty-nine witnesses appeared before the Commission. These included student leaders, other students, the university officers who had been on the ground during the incident, and a number of other members of staff. Police officers involved in the investigation also appeared. A number of self-confessed secret cult members appeared in camera. Efosa was interviewed in Ilesa Prison. The Commission also received 30 memoranda, including a comprehensive report from the University Administration on the murders, its antecedents, and the aftermath. The students presented a number of video recordings, which included the interrogations of those involved in the 7 March episode, the interrogations of Efosa, Oguaju, and the others apprehended after the 10 July episode, and some extremely gruesome photographs of the slain students.

The entire period of the Commission's sittings was full of incidents and tension. On a number of occasions, the anger of the students boiled over and there were near riots. There was a large contingent of mobile policemen inside and outside the venue, but their presence did not avert these incidents. The students appeared to respect me, and usually my appeal and that of the Students' Union leaders would help to restore order. During one particularly bad incident, when things appeared to be getting out of control, I shouted out, "I resign!" Interestingly enough, the students quietened down immediately. The members of the Commission themselves felt unsafe on that occasion, and during the subsequent afternoon session, Justice Itam publicly charged me with ensuring the good behaviour of the students.

Professor Omole's appearance before the Commission was a near disaster. He gave evidence for about two hours, to increasing clamour by the students for his arrest for the murder of their colleagues. When he finished his evidence, we had to smuggle him out through the main hall. As we got to his car, we saw a mob of stick wielding students coming towards us. We pushed him into the car and he was driven off in the nick of time.

During a sitting of the Commission, Efosa's lawyer, Mr. Atirene Wilson, presented an affidavit that had ostensibly been sworn to in the Ilesa High Court by Efosa in which he retracted his claim of Omole's involvement. The affidavit raised a lot of suspicion, since Efosa was detained in Ilesa Prison at the time when it was claimed that the affidavit had been sworn. The Commission visited the High Court where the affidavit was sworn as well as Ilesa Prison and discovered that Efosa was not the one who had sworn to the affidavit. One of the recommendations of the Commission was that the lawyer should be reported to the Bar Association. However, as with most of the Commission's recommendations, I doubt if this actually happened. On reflection, the lawyer's action was absolutely needless, since the statement by Efosa was obtained under duress. All it really achieved was to raise the possibility of collusion between Professor Omole and the lawyer, and even, by implication, with Efosa.

The Commission's report was submitted in February 2000 and was released, along with the Government's white paper, later that year. The Commission expressed its strong belief that seven named individuals had participated in the killings— Frank Idahosa (Efosa), Didi Yuletide, Kazeem Bello (Kato), and four individuals who were identified only by their nicknames or Christian names—Innocent, Athanasius, "Ochuko", and "Chunk." The last was identified as the then head of the Black Axe secret cult. The Commission also recommended the investigation of 16 other individuals, including Emeka Oguaju and the nine involved in the 7 March episode. The Panel criticised the police investigation of the case and recommended that the Inspector-General of Police should set up a special task force to take it over. I have already mentioned the recommendations concerning the Chief Magistrate who hastily tried and acquitted the 7 March culprits, as well as Efosa's lawyer. The two former Deputy VCs, the former Dean of Student Affairs, and the Registrar were criticised over aspects of the University's handling of the case and its antecedents. In the case of the Registrar, I personally believe this was unfair. In any case, the Governing Council set up a committee to examine the cases of the three who had protested against the findings and subsequently cleared all of them. The Commission was very critical of the Chief Security Officer, who was described as incompetent, and recommended that he be retired. The Director of Health Services, Dr. P.A. Odumuyiwa and his staff were commended for their handling of the victims of the attacks.

It took me several months, and a number of visits to Abuja, to obtain the Commission's report and the White Paper. Dissatisfied with the progress of the court cases, and armed with the report, I visited the Attorney-General of the Federation, Chief Bola Ige. After I had expressed my concerns over the case and highlighted the Commission's recommendations concerning its investigation, he assured me that, although the case was being prosecuted by the Osun State Attorney-General's office, his Ministry would work with that office. He sent for the Inspector-General of Police, Mr. Musiliu Smith, who agreed that he would immediately establish the recommended special task force. This he did, and a senior police officer, ACP Tonye Ibitibituwa, soon arrived in Osogbo with a team. However, in spite of the efforts of this task force, no further arrests were made. We also liaised with the Osun State Attorney-General, who assured us that his office was seriously following up the case. I must say that he did personally prosecute the case.

As I have stated, the cases against those charged in the Chief Magistrate's Court for belonging to an illegal organisation eventually came to nothing. However, we were very hopeful of a successful prosecution of the murder cases against Efosa and company. The case in the Osogbo High Court, which commenced on 9 April 2001, wound on. Evidence for the prosecution was taken from a number of students and some other witnesses. There was adjournment after adjournment. In mid-2002, the Judge hearing the case was transferred to Iwo, and the case along with it. There was a further delay while the exhibits were also subsequently taken to Iwo. To the amazement of everyone, the Judge upheld a "No Case" submission by the defence on 5 November 2002. The three accused persons were released and they subsequently disappeared. We met with the Osun State Attorney-General immediately afterwards and he expressed his amazement over the outcome of the case. He immediately gave notice of appeal and processed the relevant papers fairly quickly. I believe the appeal is still pending. However, I doubt if it will ever be possible to round up the accused individuals again.

We commemorate the murders of the five students on 10 July each year. Starting from July 2000, I would put out a release, each time concluding with the statement, "The souls of our murdered students continue to cry out for justice." On the first anniversary, we held a ceremony in Oduduwa Hall. On that occasion, the Students' Union President, Adeniyi Adenekan, took the opportunity to be publicly rude to me. I took no action because of the nature of the occasion. Soon after the murders, the students brought a proposal that the Oduduwa Hall amphitheatre be named the "Afrika Theatre," after George Iwilade. I took a proposal that the amphitheatre be named "The 10 July Theatre" to the University Senate. The proposal was rejected.

More than ten years on, I regret that the 10 July murders are gradually being forgotten. We need to remember the impact of the tragedy on the University and the nation. We also need to remember that the cry for justice for our murdered students remains unanswered.

XI

Teething Problems

I flew back to Lagos on Sunday, 18 July, arriving at Murtala Mohammed Airport at around 7.30pm. I had arranged for the Baby Friendly vehicle from the Teaching Hospital to collect me. We arrived in Ife at around 11pm. I picked up *Oga* Arigbabu from his residence in the staff quarters and we proceeded to see the Registrar, Mrs Bola Iluyomade. She gave me the letter of appointment as Acting VC which she had been asked to prepare by the Chairman of Council on the directive of the Minister. Accompanied by *Oga*, I proceeded to Awolowo Hall.

There, things appeared quiet, but students were milling around. I asked one of them where I could find the President of the Students' Union. I received no response, and, instead, we were surrounded by a small group of suspicious students. They asked what our business was. I replied, "My name is Roger Makanjuola. I have been appointed Acting VC." The response was a joyous outburst of "New VC, New VC, New VC!" As the excitement grew, we were surrounded by more and more students who insisted we should walk along with them to the Students' Union building to meet their President. The crowd, and the clamour, continued to grow as we proceeded. There were continuing shouts of "New VC" and a chant of "Roja, Roja, Roja, Roja, Roja, Roja." On the way, we met the President, 'Lanre Adeleke (Legacy). He appeared surprised, but treated me courteously and invited me to accompany him to the Students' Union building. We proceeded in the midst of the crowd of excited students. When we arrived outside the building, the President mounted the pedestal below a statue of the students who had died during a demonstration in 1980, and addressing the crowd, welcomed me. I do not remember the details of what he said, but it centred on the murders of his colleagues and allegations that the suspended VC was behind the secret cult attacks.

I replied conveying my deep sorrow over the tragic event and stated that my only objective was to restore security and normalcy to the campus. I also gave a personal undertaking that the University Administration would do everything in its power to make sure that the perpetrators were tracked down and brought to justice. We agreed that the University should be fully involved in the burials of the five murdered students the following Tuesday.

Around 3.30pm, I drove to the hospital to see the wounded students. Some had been shot, but most of them had been injured while trying to escape from the murderous assault. I saw Emeka Ojuagu, who had been arrested by the students in the aftermath of the killings and handed over to the Police after a brutal interrogation. He had been taken to the hospital by the Police and was chained to the bed. He vehemently denied involvement in the killings. However, the subsequent investigations by the Police and the Judicial Commission produced fairly weighty evidence against him.

I got to bed at around 5am the next day and still got up at 6.30am. I had slept for barely 90 minutes. I had a reputation for getting to work on time and was determined to present myself at the VC's office at 7.30am. I got there at 7.25am. There was no one there except the security staff on the ground floor, and Steven Banjo, who we all called Banjo, the VC's plain clothes security guard. Banjo got the keys so that I could be let into the office.

The office staff started drifting in from about 7.45 onwards. I went over to the house of the Deputy VC (Administration), Professor Femi Ajibola. Professor 'Bode Asubiojo was there and we discussed the situation and the impending visit of the Honourable Minister of Education that morning. The Minister, Professor 'Tunde Adeniran, had sent a message that he expected us to meet him at the University gate. We all agreed that that was not appropriate and that he should come to the VC's office. 'Bode, who knew him personally, got a message across to the Minister's staff by telephone. I went back to the office to await the Minister's arrival. I was joined by Professor Ajibola and the Registrar, Mrs. Bola Iluyomade. He arrived at about 9.30am. We went downstairs to meet him and, once the introductions had been made, he insisted that we should drive straight to the halls of residence. On the way, the Registrar expressed fear of being assaulted or even kidnapped by students. She had been briefly held and maltreated by the students some months before. I reassured her and asked her to stick by me. The entourage drove to Awolowo Hall where we had a tumultuous welcome. The Minister was taken round and shown the various rooms where the murders had taken place. During the visit, we discovered that the Registrar's fears were indeed justified. A small group of students did rain abuse on her, and, if I had not been there, she might have been assaulted.

From Awolowo Hall, we proceeded to Fajuyi Hall and thence to Oduduwa Hall, where the Minister addressed the students. I cannot remember much of what happened in Oduduwa Hall; I was too exhausted from the rigours of my trip and not having had much sleep since I returned. I do recall that Lanre Adeleke gave a rousing speech about the murders, claiming that the suspended VC was behind them. He then demanded for the recall of some eleven student leaders who had been expelled following a series of protests that had culminated in the disruption of the Convocation ceremony some years before. The Minister in his response demonstrated all his political skills. He spoke about the murders with great compassion, and assured the students that the murderers would be brought to justice. He promised that a

Judicial Commission of Enquiry would be set up to investigate the incident. He also gave an assurance that the reinstatement issue would be dealt with compassionately and that I would deal with the matter. He then invited me to address the students. All I could do was to bark out in a hoarse voice that justice would be done. The Minister departed.

I arranged to meet with the Students' Union executive later that morning and returned to the office. On getting to the office, I found a letter from the Deputy VC (Academic), Professor Akingbohungbe, in which he resigned his appointment with immediate effect. Professor Ajibola informed me that he would be also resigning, but that he would stay on until the end of the month so that I would have time to settle in and choose a successor. I have had a profound respect for Professor Ajibola since then. One Deputy VC had just unceremoniously dropped a resignation letter, while Femi had behaved decently and responsibly by staying on. Femi was extremely helpful over the next two weeks, putting me through various aspects of the administration of the University, and fulfilling his duties as a Deputy VC. I organised a small reception for him in the VC's office on the day his resignation took effect. Professor D.O. Kolawole, the Dean of Student Affairs, also submitted his resignation. Mr. Femi Idowu, the Director of Corporate Affairs, who had worked very closely with Professor Omole, had gone into hiding after the murders, believing that the students would make him a target. He came to my office early one morning with the request that he be allowed to retire with immediate effect. I agreed.

The meeting with the Students' Union took place in the major meeting room on the ground floor of the University Hall. Lanre Adeleke did much of the talking on behalf of the students. He reiterated the students' position that the suspended VC, Professor Wale Omole, and his men, were behind the murders, and that he had paid the Black Axe secret cult to carry them out. He insisted that a Judicial Panel be set up to investigate the killings. He also wanted the Students' Union, which had been banned for over a year, to be reinstated. He then raised the issue of the student leaders who had been rusticated in 1995 and requested that they be reinstated. They had been fighting a just cause against what he claimed was a repressive and corrupt administration, and, even if they deserved to be punished, they had suffered enough, having been out of the University for four years. The fourth issue raised concerned the unacceptable conditions in the halls of residence.

I responded that we were working with the Police to bring the perpetrators of the murders to justice and that I would personally speak with the Minister to ensure that a Judicial Panel was set up. I agreed to look into the cases of the rusticated students with a view to re-opening the matter and promised that I would give priority to improving the conditions under which students lived and studied. We also discussed the problem of secret cults in the University and agreed to work together to eliminate them from the campus. We agreed that, following the burials of the slain students the next day, lectures should resume on Monday, 26 July. The mobile police should remain on the campus until we felt it was safe for them to leave. They actually stayed on until the middle of September.

That evening, in the amphitheatre of Oduduwa Hall, we held a religious service for the murdered students as well as the one who had died in the road accident in the aftermath of the murders. That service was extremely moving, and it united the entire community, staff and students, in the expression of our grief. There was a special area for "dignitaries", but I sat among the students during the service, as did many others. The funerals the following day had been organised by the students. An open-air service was held on the sports field. There was a great crowd of people, with students from other universities and many representatives of trade unions. The Alumni Association had a delegation. There was a heavy media presence. Apart from me, two members of the Governing Council, Mr. 'Dimeji Arawole and Chief (Mrs.) O.O. Johnson, were there. Orations were delivered on each of the students. The one on George Iwilade (Afrika) was particularly moving. Following the service, we proceeded to the cemetery where four of the dead students were laid to rest. From there we proceeded to Iwo, the home town of George Iwilade, where he was buried amidst a great wave of grief.

As I was leaving Iwo, I was approached by a CNN team, who arranged to interview me on arrival in Ife. The interview took place in my office that evening. The interview was broadcast on CNN but I never saw it.

On Wednesday, 21 July, I called an emergency meeting of the University Senate. After informing Senate of the circumstances of my appointment as Acting VC, I gave an account of the events since my arrival. I also presented the demands of the Students' Union concerning lifting the ban on the Union, the reinstatement of the rusticated students, and welfare issues. There was a protracted discussion. Professor Bayo Lamikanra raised the issue of the perceived irregularity surrounding my appointment, which had been done without the "due process" stipulated by the University's laws. Eventually, the Senate agreed as follows:

- The Students' Union should be reinstated.
- Lectures should resume on Monday, 26 July.
- I should set up a committee to investigate the secret cult problem in the University.
- Prayers for the dead students and for the security of the University should be said during Jumat and Church services on the subsequent Friday and Sunday.

I thereafter requested for a meeting of Congregation for the afternoon of Thursday, 22 July. Congregation provides the widest forum for interaction with academic and non-academic staff of the University, since every individual with a university degree is a member. The idea was to provide a good opportunity to brief the University community about the situation on the Campus and to hold discussions with them. Unfortunately, as happened repeatedly over the next seven years, the meeting was not well attended. However, we did have useful interactions with those who came. They gave backing to the actions that had been taken since my arrival, and there was general agreement about the proposals for bringing the University back to normalcy.

That evening I experienced the first of three episodes of armed robbery attack on the university. For over a year, the campus had been suffering from repeated incursions by armed robbers, and there had been no solution to the problem. I heard over the walkie-talkie that the house of Dr. (Mrs.) Ojerinde was under attack. I requested the mobile police to go to the scene, and drove over there myself. Professor Wale Adebayo also drove over there, and we arrived at about the same time. By the time we got there, the robbers had left in Dr. Ojerinde's car, but had driven to Professor Tanwa Odebiyi's house, where they demanded entry and seized her Mercedes Benz, abandoning Dr. Ojerinde's vehicle, and then driven off again. Soon after our arrival, we heard over the radio system that the robbers were attacking Nick Igbokwe's house. The Police had joined us by then, and we all drove to Nick's house. An understandably distressed Nick and his family told us that the robbers had indeed arrived and demanded entry, but they had not gained access to the house. They shot into the house through the door and left. We spent the next hour chasing after the marauders on the Campus. Two further attacks took place the following week, with the robbers damaging doors, threatening and beating residents, and stealing money and valuables. These evil people appeared to have made the campus an open hunting ground.

Wale Adebayo was the Chairman of the Staff Quarters Security Committee, an ad-hoc sub-committee of the main Security Committee, that had been set up a year before in response to the worsening security situation in the residential areas. When I met him following the first robbery, I immediately made him Chairman of the main Security Committee. It was one of the wisest decisions I ever made. He suggested setting up a special force to combat armed robbery. The force was to be recruited from local armed guards in Ife township who had relevant experience and capability. They would be armed with shotguns, and would be provided with their own vehicle. Communication would be through the "walkie-talkie" radio communication system. A highly experienced and committed member of the University Security Department would be in control of the unit. Thus the "Cracker Unit" of the university was born. From then onwards, the problem of armed robbery on the campus rapidly abated. Armed robbers came in a few more times, but each time they were the worse off for it. Let me just say that Ife now has fewer armed robbery incidents, and fewer armed robbers, as a result of the response of the Cracker Unit. Other institutions have copied the system. Alhaji Sule Hassan and his deputy, Mr. Olafioye, organised and led this group of 25 committed and highly courageous individuals with spectacular success. This is one of the early decisions that I made, and one of the most significant. As you will see later, they even had a major preventive influence on secret cultism because the students were afraid of them.

Professor Wale Omole's life was under threat, presumably from the students, and so he kept away from the campus. He and his wife, Sade, went through a terrible time. The danger was not imaginary. Following a telephone conversation during the previous week, on Sunday, 25 July I travelled down to Ibadan and met him in the Premier Hotel. He briefed me on important issues concerning the administration of the campus. Amongst other things, he was concerned about the continuity of some important development projects he had started. He was particularly concerned that his innovative Central Science Laboratory project be completed. One vivid remark stuck in my mind when we were talking about the leadership of the Laboratory. "I put Professor Ako-Nai in charge of this. However, I know you will want to put your own man there," he said. I knew Kwashi Ako-Nai quite well, and had a great admiration for him. My response was that, "He is a good man for the job. I will keep him on." He appeared amazed.

One of the characteristics of Nigerians is that, when we are placed in new positions, we tend not to trust our predecessors. Thus, the first thing a Nigerian new broom does when he takes up a post is to sweep everyone out. My decision to keep Kwashi was absolutely right. He organised the Central Science Laboratory extremely effectively. He was totally committed to the project, and highly capable. He became one of my closest friends.

Lectures resumed on Monday, 26 July without any problem. The atmosphere was peaceful. I guess everyone, staff and students, was relieved to be getting back to normal activities. There was still some tension, because many of the students, in particular, were afraid of a repeat attack, particularly since some of the Black Axe members had been arrested and some tortured. We kept the mobile police on the campus for a further eight weeks, and their presence further calmed the situation and made us feel safer. Even the students, who have a proverbial antipathy towards the Police, wanted them to stay.

In the meantime, we continued to liaise with the Commissioner of Police over the arrest and prosecution of individuals mentioned in the murder case.

I spoke with the Pro-Chancellor, retired Justice A.N. Aniagolu, soon after my arrival. In the aftermath of the murders, Council members were considered to be at risk from attack by angry students. On reflection, this appears to have been rather far-fetched, but various irrational presumptions were made in its support, e.g., they were close to Wale Omole, the suspended VC, whom the Students' Union claimed to be behind the attacks. However, towards the end of that first week, Justice Aniagolu insisted that the Council must meet, and we agreed on 27 July. Because of the perceived security risks, the meeting was arranged to take place in the Chancellor's Lodge, and was not publicised. The meeting was attended by all the members, except Professor Akingbohungbe, who had resigned as Deputy VC (Academic).

The Pro-Chancellor expressed his deep dismay over the murders. He stated that he was in Abuja when he learnt of the incident, and issued a press release which the Nigeria Television Authority had distorted in its news bulletin later that day. He briefed Council on the circumstances of my appointment. Professor Ajibola then provided a detailed report on the murders and their immediate aftermath. He expressed some concern over the role of the Commissioner of Police who appeared to be working in a manner that was likely to hinder communication and cooperation between the student body and the University administration. I briefed Council on developments since my arrival. I expressed grave concern over the incident in March that year when a group of students had been apprehended with guns and other weapons in their possession but were subsequently discharged and acquitted by the Chief Magistrate, accompanied by an order to destroy the evidence.

Council reiterated its dismay and deep distress over the murders. It directed me to continue to liaise closely with the Police to ensure that the perpetrators were brought to book. I was to facilitate cooperation between the Police and the students and also convey to the Assistant Inspector-General of Police in the Zone Council's concern over the manner in which the March incident had been handled. Council expressed dismay over the distortion of the Pro-Chancellor's release by the NTA and directed that the correct release be widely circulated. It then issued a special release on the incident. A sum of ₦50,000 was approved for the families of each of the murdered students. It also approved a University scholarship for one member of each family. A ₦1 million Trust Fund was to be established to provide a scholarship fund in memory of the dead students. This actually never happened. When the matter was raised at the next meeting, Council agreed that the Fund should be launched at the beginning of the following semester. However, by the next semester the Council had been dissolved. Council closed the business of the day by accepting "with regret" the resignations of the two Deputy VCs.

As the University gradually returned to normal, I continued to meet with various committees, groups, and individuals who were considered to be in a position to help or advise me. I may have overdone it with respect to some individuals. I felt that if I went out of my way to meet with individuals who were perceived as having influence, or who considered themselves to be influential, they might be more willing to help and support me—the whole idea was of openness.

Some of these so-called influential individuals misinterpreted this relatively humble approach as weakness or dependence on my part. I once went to a senior Professor's house one morning to seek his advice. Within a few days, I heard that he was openly boasting that he could summon me any time and I would come running to his house!

The reception that I got from the staff unions was, by and large, lukewarm. The then Chairman of ASUU was Dr. Idowu Awopetu. During meetings with him and his executive, hostility towards me was palpable; this hostility continued until I left office seven years later. We do get on quite well now though. I believe ASUU felt that my appointment was unfair and against the laid-down procedures of the University. However, the University laws do not make provision for the most unusual circumstances in which I was appointed Acting VC. The other staff unions were reasonably supportive, at least initially.

My relationship with the Students' Union gradually became productive, at least during Legacy's time. They had made it clear from the start that they would cooperate with me for as long as they considered it in their interest—"No permanent friend, no permanent enemy, only permanent interests." We continued to work together on the secret cult problem, and the programme we set up certainly would not have worked without them.

We continued to liaise with the Commissioner of Police over the arrest and prosecution of the murderers. The students had set up a special committee to prosecute the perpetrators under an individual who was clearly psychopathic; he used his position to persecute all and sundry, including some innocent individuals. The students drew up a list of suspects and their whereabouts; we passed this information on to the Police. We also provided logistic support to the Police, particularly transportation and transportation expenses. The outcome of the investigation and trial has been outlined earlier.

The student body is the major factor in the success of any campaign against secret cults. If the students decide to eliminate secret cults on any campus, then the cults will be eliminated. Without their active cooperation and participation, nothing will happen. Following the receipt of the report of the Committee that I had set up under the chairmanship of Professor Funso Sonaiya, we drew up a programme to deal with the problem. The programme had three inter-related thrusts—preventive, rehabilitative, and punitive. After the 10 July murders, the Federal Government provided a special fund to all the universities to combat the secret cult problem. Ife got ₦15 million; the others got ₦10 million each. We actually presented a budget of ₦18.7 million to the Governing Council and it approved the additional ₦3.7 million from the University's own resources. I mention this figure because subsequent Students' Union executives headed by Adenekan and later Olawoyin accused me of stealing the ₦15 million. I informed them that the correct figure was ₦18.7 million!

The preventive aspect of our programme included orientation on cultism and its dangers aimed at the students and the wider community. We paid particular attention to the most vulnerable group, the younger students, providing information on how the cults went about recruiting members, and of their horrific practices once any person had fallen into their trap. We also provided improved sporting and recreational facilities as alternative social outlets.

We embarked on a programme of renunciations. Secret cult members who wished to get out of the trap were encouraged to approach Deans, Heads of Department, members of the University administration, the various religious groups, and the Students' Union. Absolute confidentiality was guaranteed, and a variety of counselling services were made available depending on the wishes of the individual concerned. I personally dealt with a number of cases and referred them to churches, our clinical psychology unit and, in one case, to the Muslim Community.

Wale Adebayo and, later, Dr. G.O. Babalola, after he was appointed Acting Dean of Student Affairs, coordinated joint activities of the University's Security Services with the Students' Union to identify those cult members who did not wish to renounce their membership, and to combat their activities. We used to hand them over to the Police. However, once I was convinced, I would suspend them from the University and make it clear that they would not be welcomed back. Unfair? Not in compliance with a fair hearing? But I had to deal with the problem, and be seen to deal with it, ruthlessly. We succeeded.

From being in the forefront of the secret cult problem, OAU became one of the most cult-free universities in the country. We did not totally eliminate secret cults from the University, but we certainly achieved a drastic reduction. Whatever secret cult activity remained, it was at a minimum and operating strictly underground. There are universities in this country where secret cults operate openly, and where they even play football matches against each other. When the Federal government released the special fund to combat secret cults in universities, one secret cult demanded that the VC of their university give them a share—after all, the money was meant for the secret cults! Not in Ife.

XII

Industrial Unrest

The tension in the campus gradually dissipated, peace returned and the academic programme progressed. Initially, I combined the duties of the two Deputy VCs who had resigned with mine. The duties of a Deputy VC (Administration) largely involve the supervision of the support services. In the past, the Registrar handled these. I personally believe that there was never any real justification for taking those responsibilities away from that office. If academics had to take over the administration and supervision of areas such as maintenance services and security, then this was a reflection of the poor capabilities of the officers in the Registry and the maintenance services rather than the need for an overhaul of the system. When I started work, I found the various units under the portfolio of the Deputy VC (Administration) reasonably well run, and so I was able to cope fairly well with them. The Director of the Division of Works and Maintenance Services, Alhaji Bakare, was fairly effective and highly responsible. Professor Adebayo effectively ran the Security Services. However, the duties of the Deputy VC (Academic) were a different matter. I needed someone in that position quickly. The then Chairman of the

Committee of Deans was Professor Anthony Elujoba. By virtue of his position, I worked closely with him and I got to know and appreciate his administrative capabilities. He knew the academic system of the University inside out. I believed he would make an excellent Deputy VC (Academic) and so I went to see him one Sunday morning about proposing him for the job. As I finished my spiel, his wife came down the stairs and he informed her of my request. Both were delighted, and Tony there and then accepted, with a sincere undertaking to put everything he had into the task. We agreed that a meeting of the University Senate should be called and his name be put forward for election. I went home a happy man.

Later that day, Tony came to my house, accompanied by Professor Wale Akinsola, his close friend. Professor Akinsola was the nephrologist who had so successfully headed the Hospital's renal team. Tony reminded me that the University laws stipulated that two candidates should be nominated and that Senate would then elect one of the two. I was worried, what if I put up another candidate and Tony lost? I wanted Tony. I thought for a minute and then naively hatched a way out — "Let us nominate you and Professor Akinsola and on the day of the election, Professor Akinsola can withdraw." I swear I did not think of the implications of this. What I had proposed actually amounted to an attempt to subvert the laws of the University. All I wanted was a good and loyal man by my side. I maintain to this day that, at the time, I did not really appreciate the implications of my action. If I had, I would never have done it. However, the three of us agreed on my proposal.

On the 3 August, the University Senate held a special meeting to elect the Deputy VC (Academic). The two nominations were read out and immediately afterwards, Wale Akinsola announced his withdrawal from the contest. There was an uproar. The members declared that the election could not take place unless there were two candidates. I recall that Professor Olutiola declared, "You cannot deprive me of my right to vote." Now we were back to square one. The three of us met thereafter and agreed that both candidates should be put forward again, but this time to follow due process. Senate met again two weeks later. To my surprise, Wale Akinsola won by three votes. I still feel bad about this incident to this day. It reflected badly on me, but what I regretted even more was the hurt that it caused to Tony and his family. I met his wife, a very delightful lady, soon afterwards and told her how truly sorry I was about what I had done to their family. Wale Akinsola did turn out to be a very competent Deputy VC.

The Dean of Student Affairs, Professor D.O. Kolawole, had resigned along with the two Deputy VCs. Initially, I personally handled matters concerning the students, while looking around for a suitable Dean. I raised the matter with Dipo Fasina in his house one evening. At that time, Dipo was the National President of ASUU, but that was not why I sought his advice. Dipo has been a friend for many years, we were in King's College together and when the staff cricket team was established in the University, he became a member. After I was appointed Acting VC, I consulted him regularly. I found his advice extremely valuable. He was, and is, a completely honest, decent person with a great knowledge of the university system and its politics. He was greatly maligned by many, especially in Government circles, but, in fact, he is a scrupulously honest individual who wants the best for the university system and for the country. Of course, he is a politician, but his decency overrides all that. I rejected the first person he suggested and he then suggested Dr. Gbolahan Babalola. I had known Dr. Babalola (*Bablo*) for many years. We were both active members of the Staff Club. We agreed he would do the job well. He related well with the students and had a good understanding of their needs. I drove over to *Bablo*'s house and offered him the job. He readily agreed, with the proviso that I would back his efforts to promote the welfare of the students. Since he was not yet a professor, he couldn't be made a Dean and so I appointed him Acting Dean of Student Affairs.

Bablo has a great depth of knowledge of the students and of their politics. He also related to them extremely well, and in such a manner that he did not lose their respect. His response to their emergencies was instantaneous and he had the patience and the stamina to spend long hours dealing with their problems. Students, or at least student leaders, are very verbose, and I often lost patience during negotiations with them. *Bablo* was infinitely patient. I believe the students also knew that he had their interests at heart and was absolutely committed to their welfare. He was one of the closest associates I had. He, like many of our alumni, are truly committed and extremely proud of their alma mater. Some of the academic staff felt he allowed the students to be "over-familiar." This was unavoidable at that time, because the student body was so suspicious of us. He also enjoyed his beer, much to the chagrin of the Moslems and "born again" Christian community. *Bablo* got to work, and gained not only the trust but also the respect of the majority of the students, including the Students' Union Executive. I left him to it, confident that he would deal with things effectively and, more importantly, that I would not have to keep looking over my shoulder to see what he was up to. With *Bablo*, I only had to get involved when things were really difficult and he needed some support.

A lot of work was involved, and we had to look for a deputy for *Bablo*. Again, we were fortunate. *Bablo* suggested Dr. Yemisi Obilade, a lecturer in the Faculty of Education. She was also an alumna, and a firebrand. Along with Dr. Toyin Fasina, she founded the organisation Women Against Rape, Sexual Harassment and Sexual Exploitation (WARSHE). At a time when Gender Equity was a foreign concept in the University, she and Toyin were already in the forefront of the fight. She brooked no nonsense from anyone. Outside the student body itself, no one had such a deep knowledge and understanding of students and student politics. She accepted the Vice-Deanship, and she and *Bablo* were a great team. Her firmness with the students stood her in good stead. Once she had taken her stand, the students knew that no amount of manipulation or even violence would shift her. Dr. Babalola's promotion to Professor came through in 2004. I made him substantive Dean immediately afterwards.

In August 1999, the Federal Government sent visitation panels to all its universities. Ours arrived at the beginning of September. Prior to its arrival, the Governing Council, in considering its terms of reference, had expressed concern over one term of reference, viz. to ascertain whether there were any financial irregularities or incidences of financial mismanagement in the University during the five-year period covered by the visitation. The Council requested me to investigate a number of projects over which the staff unions, especially ASUU, had made claims of financial mismanagement. I carried out a fairly straightforward appraisal of these projects. I hired a Quantity Surveyor that I had used to investigate some projects in the hospital when I was CMD. Her valuations of quantities and rates were then compared with those on the contract. She also remeasured the actual quantities. I supplemented the investigation with information from the files. We did conclude that a number of awards had been overpriced by up to one-third. When I presented the report to the Chairman of the Governing Council, he chose not to table it. The Visitation Panel raised the matter in its report, but nothing ever came of it. The Panel spent over a month with us, occupying much of our time, as well as the University's resources. It produced a lengthy report, followed by a Government White Paper, but most of its contents were never implemented, possibly never read at all. Indeed, when the next Visitation Panel arrived in 2005, they came with a large number of copies of the 1999 White Paper that they wanted us to sell through the bookshop.

The major crises we faced during that "Acting Administration" were over industrial actions and communal problems. The first industrial action was by the Non-Academic Staff Union of Educational and Associated Institutions (NASU) and the Senior Staff Association of Nigerian Universities (SSANU), in November, 1999. I forget what the problem was. All I remember was that it was a national industrial action. They went on strike, leaving all the support services unmanned. For years their practice during industrial actions was to withdraw the supply of electricity and water. They would even sabotage the installations to ensure that, even if the University succeeded in bringing people in to operate them, this would not be possible. In any case, they believed that no one else could operate these systems. Needless to say, they would allow Bursary staff to come in to process salaries when due. Just as with the Health Care system, the University staff were confident about being paid their salaries even when they were on strike. In the past, they had even negotiated with the University Administration for the provision of electricity and water supply during strikes, provided that those who came in to provide these services were paid extra. We met with the two unions, but could not obtain any concessions unless we agreed to "compensate" those who would provide the services. I refused to pay such "compensation." The strike lasted for two weeks, during which there was much suffering among members of the University community, including the striking workers and their families.

SSANU and NASU went on strike again on 23 February 2000. This time, it was a local dispute. The academic staff had been awarded a special allowance by the Government for the administration of examinations. Subsequently, the laboratory technologists had also been awarded an Examination Administration Allowance. SSANU and NASU claimed that they too were entitled to this allowance, since they were also involved in the administration of examinations. They stated that without their input, examinations could not be held. The arguments went to ludicrous lengths. For instance, they asserted that the tanker attendants were entitled to an allowance because they delivered water to the halls of residence during examinations. We were anxious to avoid any disruption in view of our recent history. We were also conscious that the examinations were approaching. We put forward a compromise to the effect that non-teaching staff who were directly involved in examinations, such as the staff of the Examinations Office, should receive the allowance. This was rejected, and the two unions embarked on an all-out strike. They abandoned the water works, power house, and other electrical installations. The water supply ceased immediately, and once there was an outage from the public power supply, electricity supply ceased because the power could not be switched back on after it was restored from the public supply. Refuse collection also ceased, and garbage accumulated all over the campus, particularly in the halls of residence. You can imagine what it was like with 23,000 students in overcrowded hostels without power, water, or sanitation. Things were desperate. The University Administration, comprising the Acting VC; the Deputy VC (Academic), Wale Akinsola; the Chairman, Committee of Deans, Tony Elujoba; the Registrar, Bola Iluyomade; the Librarian, Michael Afolabi; and the Bursar, Mrs. Aladekomo, met repeatedly with the two unions to try to resolve the impasse or, at least, to obtain some concessions on water and power supply. The Chairman of SSANU at the time was Mr. M.O. Afolabi, a thoroughly bellicose character, very different from his namesake the Librarian, who was, and continues to be, a truly decent person. The NASU Chairman was Mr. Niyi Akinnibi, seemingly more reasonable than his SSANU counterpart, but in fact equally malignant. They would not budge. On one occasion, during a meeting with the unions, I burst into tears. They were unmoved.

On the first night of the strike, I went secretly to the water works. I found that the clear water tank, where the processed water was stored, was full, and switched on the high lift pump that sent water to the campus. It worked! Water started emptying from the tank and flowing into the halls and around the campus. Unfortunately, I miscalculated the emptying rate—if the tank was not recharged continuously, it actually emptied within about three-quarters of an hour. I left the pump on and, feeling very happy with myself, went for a beer in the Staff Club. By the time I returned, the tank was empty and the system was full of air. It would have to be primed before it would function again, and, because of a leak in the system, a substantial amount of water would be required for this. The following Sunday, I decided to try to sort out the problem. The day before, I had run the low lift pump that sent raw water through the system and filled the processed water tank again. I had not employed any chemicals, but hoped that the filtration system would at least make the water clean enough for washing, if not for drinking. *Oga* Arigbabu and I went over to Alhaji Bakare's house and requested his advice. He reluctantly gave the advice, but was pessimistic about our chances of success. He was very frightened, and told us that the two unions had threatened to use *juju* against him if he helped us. He also warned us that a curse had been invoked on the water works so that any person who entered the premises would die. We left, and spent two hours trying to get the pump to work. We were armed with shotguns, because the unions had sent out death threats against anyone who tried to run the water and power systems. While there, Professor Sola Ogedengbe arrived. He claimed to be an expert on the water system, but when we invited him to sort out the problem, it was obvious that he had no clue. He had more head knowledge than practical knowledge. There are many like him in the university system. Later, Professor Ogedengbe reported that we had threatened him with guns. As I stated earlier, it was true that we were armed, but we never pointed the guns at him, and how he concluded that we threatened him is beyond me.

We returned to Alhaji Bakare's house to find him being carried into an ambulance. He had collapsed soon after we left. A doctor had been called who had not found anything physically wrong with him, and subsequent investigations at the Health Centre also could not provide an explanation for his condition. His belief in *juju* had precipitated the collapse. Either that, or *juju* actually works! Anyway, Alhaji Bakare gave us no more help or advice, and requested that I stay away from his home.

I requested the Hospital to provide water to the halls through its tanker. The unions waylaid the tanker and it had to turn back. One of our contractors, Prince Adewa, also tried to provide water through his company's tanker. He was waylaid in the junior staff quarters and the tyres of his car were slashed. That tanker also had to turn back.

Things were grim. Two weeks into the strike, I went to see the State Governor in Osogbo to seek his help with the water supply. The Governor was not available but his deputy saw me. This was my first meeting with Otunba Iyiola Omisore, the

Deputy Governor at that time. Without hesitation, he agreed to organise water supply to the University through a number of Government tankers. He also got in touch with the Commandant of the Military Cantonment in Ede, who agreed to supply the University through their 33,000-litre tanker. He also offered technical help from Ede Water Works if we needed it. Otunba Omisore is a controversial figure. All I do know is that he helped the University very effectively when we were in serious trouble. The tanker services he provided came in every day, and provided water mainly to the halls of residence. The tankers were able to come in through the main gates unhindered, probably because the striking members of staff feared the wrath of the students. However, things still remained very difficult. There was still no electricity and the garbage continued to accumulate, and the examinations were approaching.

I called a special meeting of Senate on 27 February 2000 to brief it on the situation. There was tremendous hostility over the manner in which I had handled the situation—yes, it was all directed at me. The major source of resentment that I picked up was that we had offered to pay some of the non-academic staff the Examination Administration Allowance. They appeared to see this as an acknowledgment that non-academic staff were involved in academic duties and also as an infringement of an award that had been made exclusively for academic staff. There were also deeper sources of resentment that were more personal. The members of Senate were understandably furious over the behaviour of the striking members of staff and the suffering by the community as a result of the withdrawal of water and electricity. Under a "Point of Information," Dr. Ayo Salami, a representative of Congregation and a university politician, got up at one stage and stated, "Mr. Vice-Chancellor, I put it to you that you are incompetent." I replied that this was a rhetorical question that required no answer. He shouted, "It is not a rhetorical question. I demand an answer." Professor M.S. Akanni of the Department of Chemistry was also extremely furious. However, he employed more civil language. He was subsequently to make very valuable contributions as Head of the Chemistry Department and, even more importantly, as Coordinator of the Pre-degree Programme. At the end of the increasingly heated debate, I started to summarise. Professor Bayo Lamikanra, who had also been highly, and rudely, critical during the meeting, stood up and said, "There is no need for you to summarise. I shall summarise for you. You should restore light and water. We don't care how you do it. Go and do it." The meeting ended. I walked out of the hall in an atmosphere of hostility from almost all the members of Senate. This was the lowest point I ever reached during my seven years as VC. My gloom evaporated when, an hour later, Bayo Amole came into my house and said, "Roger, what can I do to help?" That truly encouraged me, and Bayo became the main individual who coordinated the tanker supply from the State Government and the Military. Bayo proved indispensable throughout my administration. He is also one of my closest friends.

Senate had already decided that the semester examinations should be held and had made contingency plans for this. The support services normally provided by the administrative staff, including the distribution of question papers, would be provided by academic staff, under the direction of the Deans. Anticipating trouble when the examinations began, I asked for, and obtained, a small detachment of policemen, who entered the campus on the evening of Friday, 25 February. The next morning, the students held a congress at which they resolved that they did not want any policemen on the campus, and that their presence should be resisted. Hearing of this, I decided that the policemen should withdraw. They could not have done much anyway. They were not the mobile policemen that I had requested for, and they were too few. On the same Saturday that the police withdrew, members of the two striking unions went on the rampage, assaulting members of academic staff in particular. One of those they attacked was *Bablo*. The students were enraged by the attack on their Dean and went out to seek the perpetrators. They got the main culprit, 'Bimbo Awopileda, and drove him off in a bus. I managed to stop the bus, in which Bimbo was cowering in obvious fear for his life. I lied to the students that were holding Bimbo, that he was not the guilty one. I managed to persuade them to let me take him away. I have never seen anyone so terrified before or since. If I had not persuaded the students to release him to me, heaven knows what might have happened to him—they were truly incensed. That weekend was completely chaotic. Apart from their increasing hostility towards the members of SSANU and NASU, the students had also become hostile to ASUU. They saw them as having been, in part, responsible for provoking the strike by antagonising SSANU and NASU through resisting the grant to them of the examination allowance. During their congress on 26 February, the chant went up, "ASUU is the problem." After that congress in the amphitheatre, a mob of students came across Drs. Awopetu and Ukponmwan and tried to hold them hostage. *Bablo* and I had to stand between them and eventually conducted the two ASUU members to a classroom, after which the students dispersed. I remember that the two reacted very differently to the situation. Dr. Idowu Awopetu was extremely angry. Dr. Otas Ukponmwan, on the other hand, was petrified.

The two unions employed violence and threats to prosecute their strike. They particularly targeted academic staff, and two professors were physically assaulted. One morning, I returned from a trip to Ilesa to be informed that the Deputy VC (Academic) Wale Akinsola, had been taken hostage. The Chairmen of SSANU and NASU, along with some other thugs, had left a joint congress and proceeded to his office, and had forced him to accompany them to the sports field. I was furious at the news, and went straight to the Sports Center, where I found Wale sitting on the stadium steps, surrounded by thugs and being harangued by Mr. Afolabi, the SSANU Chairman. I went over to Wale, told him to get up and walked off with him. They did not follow us; they must have seen how angry I was.

The behaviour of the two striking unions continued to worsen. They had used violence and threats to great effect in the past and they believed that this was the way to achieve their ends. They saw the academic staff as their enemies, particularly after Senate decided that it would go ahead with the examinations in spite of the strike. The threats were open. I met with the NASU and SSANU leadership early one morning and obtained a promise that the threats and intimidation would cease. Instead, that same morning, 29 February, they brought a masquerade to their congress at the Sports Centre. ASUU also held a congress that morning and at their request, I went down to address them. The ASUU members expressed their concerns over the threats against them and about the masquerade on the sports field. I gave them an assurance that they would not be attacked and returned to my office. An hour later, I received a radio message that the striking workers, accompanied by the masquerade, had gone to the ASUU congress and attacked them. I ran down to the scene at the Humanities lecture theatre, accompanied by a TV crew who filmed the whole incident. I found that the majority of the ASUU members had fled, although a few still remained. The masquerade was dancing around and the rest of the mob was armed with whips. I was enraged. I grabbed a whip from the hand of one of the attackers and started chasing them, whipping them right, left and centre. I also chased after the masquerade, who jumped over a hedge and ran off. I actually saw his underpants as he jumped over—they were blue. The NTA crew filmed the whole incident. Fortunately, what was shown on the TV that evening was heavily edited. It showed me chasing after the mob and the masquerade, but did not include some of the strong language that I used.

We knew that the power house was intact. The supply from NEPA (the public supply) was on. What was required was to switch the system on. This was a procedure that required some skill. For reasons that are not yet clear to me, the general opinion was that only the power house staff could do it. I did not believe this, and this opinion was bolstered when the Head of the Department of Electronic and Electrical Engineering, Professor Adegboyega, came to my house and said that they could switch the power back on. I requested him to get a team ready. The unions suspected we might try, and they put a guard around the power house. It was rumoured that they were armed, but, although I did see these guards at the power house gate, I could not be sure whether they were armed or not. I received many warnings not to go near the power house. One story had it that the installation had been sabotaged so that it would explode if anyone tampered with it. I remember in particular that Juliet Dixon, a close friend, went down on her knees, begging me not to go near the power house. They had also put various items of *juju* around the premises. We had planned to go in on the day after the contingent of police were brought into the campus, but had to postpone it when the police were driven away by the students.

In the first week of March 2000, the communal crisis between the Ife and the Modakeke communities flared up again. The security situation in the town rapidly deteriorated. On the afternoon of Sunday, 5 March, I passed by the power house and noted that the picketing union members had left. I took the opportunity to destroy all the *juju* they had strewn around, much to the horror of onlookers. One item was particularly gruesome —a clay pot containing a dead rat, feathers, palm oil, ashes, and dried blood. I went over to Professor Adegboyega's house and requested him to get his team ready to restore the electrical power that night. We agreed to go in at 12 midnight. Before that time, I went to the house of Mr. Abisa, the head of the electrical unit, with Dr. Komolafe. Mr. Abisa briefed us on what to do. He was very scared of the repercussions if the unions heard he had been helping us, and could not come to the power house with us. We went in shortly after midnight. The team comprised Dr. Komolafe, Dr. Omoigui, Professor Mike Faborode, who was to be my successor as VC, and myself. A team of Crackers, security men employed by us to combat the wave of armed robberies in the campus, accompanied us. We broke the locks of the power house door and Dr. Komolafe got to work. He followed Mr. Abisa's instructions, but nothing happened. In despair, I drove back to Mr. Abisa's house along with Mike Faborode. Mr. Abisa reluctantly agreed to accompany us to fix the system. On the way back, we saw that the lights were on! Dr. Komolafe had initially forgotten to switch on the main incoming breaker switch. We then went round switching on all the sub-stations that the striking workers had switched off. The myth was broken—we could run the power system. And we continued to do so thereafter. We even had a maintenance team for the distribution system comprising Dr. Ladi Osasona and Dr. Omoigui. They carried out a number of repairs to the low tension and high tension lines. I, with a number of others, became an expert at running the power house. The unions' power over electricity supply was broken.

While power had been restored, the water situation was still very bad. The tanker supply was limited, and the examinations were fast approaching. I decided to try once more to get the water works functioning. I approached Otunba Omisore, who ordered the staff of Ede Water Works to help. We agreed that they should come in on a Friday evening. I also arranged for one of Osun State's water tankers to come in with a full load so that we could prime the high lift pump. Interestingly enough, that morning the Chairman of NASU had offered to restore water supply if we would compensate the staff involved. I told him I would think about it. That afternoon, Mr. Afolabi, the Librarian, went to Ede to bring the technical crew that was to help. They stayed in his house until we were ready to go. At about 11pm, I took them to the water works. The tanker was waiting there. Mr. Adamu, a retired member of the water unit was also with us. The crew first ran the water treatment plant and filled up the clear water tank. We then opened up one of the high lift pumps and primed it with water from the tanker. When we switched the pump on, it failed to pump anything. We tried again, this time with more water. We switched on again, and there was an explosion as the rubber gasket flew off in a burst of water. The loss of the gasket was bad, but we knew we had got the pump working. We replaced the gasket and restarted the pump. Gradually, the pressure built up and water started flowing to the campus. The Ede crew stayed with us for a week, during which I and a few others learnt how to run the system. Another expert was brought in to show us how to run the backwash system for cleaning the filtration tanks. From then until the strike ended, the water and power supply systems were run by our small group.

As for the refuse, the Dean of Student Affairs organised some evacuation in and around the halls of residence through some local contractors. This partly alleviated the sanitation problem.

In all future strikes by the non-academic staff, we were able to run both power and water systems. However, NASU and SSANU did not accept that their power had been broken. They made one further attempt to assert their power through the use of violence a year later. Violence appeared to have been rewarded, and, in accordance with the psychological theories of learning, if violence is rewarded, in other words positively reinforced, then violence will be much more likely to be employed in the future. I guess they felt that they had not been violent enough the first time around, and that they needed to exert more force in what amounted to our final engagement.

While we were battling with our problems in the university, the communal crisis between Ife and Modakeke worsened. Academic activities had come to a stop. We had to request for a contingent of mobile policemen to protect the University from the warring factions. In the town, there were pitched battles, especially in the "no man's land" between the two territories, over which each group claimed ownership. This war zone included the area just outside the University gates. A student was shot in the hand at the gate. On a number of occasions, these battles occurred just outside the gates, into which the mobile policemen, protecting us inevitably got drawn. I witnessed one such gunfight at close quarters. On that occasion, I was truly impressed by the apparent fearlessness of the "Mopol." Members of both communities were targeted in the town, and houses perceived as belonging to their opponents were attacked and set on fire. The campus became a refuge for those living in the town who were in fear of their lives.

Large numbers of university staff and students living in the town, most of whom did not belong to either side, were displaced. They fled in terror. Many had to leave their property behind in the burning houses. They would arrive on the campus with their families, all of them in distress, sometimes with only the clothes they had on. We set up a committee to accommodate our displaced colleagues. I put Dr. Wale Rotimi in charge. Day and night he would organise places for them to stay. We used the Postgraduate Hall, the chalets of the Conference Centre, and every residence that was free within the campus. Things were difficult for them, but at least they were safe, and we managed to put a roof over every head. Members of the University community also, on their own, accommodated many of the refugees. The students readily rose to the occasion and housed every one of their displaced colleagues in the halls of residence.

The President, Chief Olusegun Obasanjo, visited Osun State at the height of the crisis and I sought an audience with him in order to explain the plight of our staff and students and obtain his help. He received me early one morning in Osogbo, with great courtesy. After I had briefed him on the situation, he advised me to approach the National Disaster Relief Agency. He then asked my opinion on some individuals who had been nominated for the position of Pro-Chancellor of the University. I gave a very blunt appraisal of the nominees. The advice stuck in his mind; because he reminded me of my advice and of the blunt language I had employed during a meeting in Abuja five years later.

Members of the University community come from all over the country. However, it must be recorded that a few of those who were members of the two warring sides, who were actively involved in the "war," were members of staff. A lecturer in the Department of Urban and Regional Planning was caught by the Police carrying a substantial cache of arms and ammunition in his car. He was shown on the television, sitting on the floor, manacled and surrounded by the weapons he had been carrying. He spent time in prison custody, but was eventually released, I presume as part of the settlement of the communal crisis. He returned to the campus, and, to my relief, requested for sabbatical leave, which I granted immediately. I would have expected that this individual would have used the opportunity of the sabbatical to seek employment elsewhere, but he did not, and returned to the University after his sabbatical.

We met repeatedly with representatives of both sides of the communal crisis on the campus. I do not believe the meetings did much to reduce the enmity between the two sides, but we did at least establish that the campus should remain a place of safety and refuge for all persons, including members of the warring factions. Towards the end of active hostilities, I made available a venue on the campus for peace meetings between the two communities, with neutral members of the University featuring prominently among the peacemakers. I was personally involved in some of those meetings.

On 5 March, the body of a young lady was brought into the campus by individuals who were never identified but were most certainly students of the University. The body was taken to the Students' Union building and lay in state outside. Large numbers of students gathered at the scene, and the Students' Union President, Adeniyi Adenekan, presided over the event from a podium. He claimed that the corpse was that of a student of the University. The Dean, Student Affairs, went to the scene and arranged for the body to be removed to the mortuary in the hospital. Adenekan, of whom you will read more later, capitalised on the incident. He presided over a congress that pronounced a one-week period of mourning and the postponement of the forthcoming examinations. The University Senate decided that the examinations should go ahead, but the students did succeed in violently disrupting them for the first two days. The examinations finally went ahead on 9 March. We soon discovered that the dead lady was not a student, but by then the emotions of the students had been whipped up. The boycott of lectures and postponement of examinations were never approved by the University Senate, nevertheless the University was presented with a fait accompli. We set up a Panel to find out the facts of the matter, but we never did identify the culprits who had brought the body into the campus. We had strong suspicions that student leaders may have been behind it. The real tragedy is that this young lady, who had been shot in the communal cross-fire, had died so needlessly, and unscrupulous individuals had taken advantage of the tragedy for their own ends.

On 8 May, a medical student, 'Seni Osunade, was kidnapped at Sabo, while waiting for transport to the hospital. He was never seen again. I later learnt that he was taken to a site on the eastern side of the township and murdered within a few minutes of being taken away. Seni was from Tonkere, a village that the Ifes saw as allied to the Modakekes. We got to work on the case and a culprit was arrested, but the witness who was with 'Seni when he was kidnapped was in fear of his life and refused to make the identification. Today, that murderer is still on the loose and maybe working just outside the University gate.

As mentioned earlier, the University had gradually ground to a virtual standstill. On 10 May, Senate formally closed the University. We did not resume until the end of June.

One day at the height of the crisis, I foolishly drove to the Police headquarters in town along the main road, the western end of which was in the war zone. I was shot at but escaped unscathed. I reported the matter to the Area Commandeer on arrival at the Police Station. The report is probably what led to the publication in the *Sunday Punch* of 7 May 2000, with the headline, "OAU VC, Bishop, shot." The article stated that I had been shot, along with the Anglican Bishop of Ile-Ife Diocese and one Dennis M. Carpenter, a "white man." The publication went on to state that we had all been admitted to the Intensive Care Unit of the hospital in a critical condition and that the doctors and nurses were battling to save our lives. My family heard the news before I did and were extremely distressed. The Minister of Education, Professor 'Tunde Adeniran, was one of the many individuals who sent people to Ife to check on the story. I arrived in Abuja later that day and he was incredulous, though quite relieved to see me. I met the reporter who wrote this article a few weeks later. He admitted that he had had no firm evidence for his claim but was not remorseful about the totally unfounded story.

Mr. 'Layi Alabi, a close friend, had a very successful motor business, which was based in the war zone. His residence is behind the business. He was a close friend. Although he did not belong to either of the warring ethnic groups, he had received several threats and, on a number of occasions, had had to fire warning shots to drive off various combatant groups. The house next to his was burnt to the ground during one attack. However, he was determined to stay put. One Saturday afternoon, Oga Arigbabu phoned me to say that 'Layi was once more under attack and in grave danger. We decided to go and rescue him. We drove out of the main gate and onto the Old Ede Road leading towards his house. Half-way along, we realised we were in the middle of a fire fight. Bullets were flying and those caught up in the crossfire were either lying flat on the ground or crawling to safety. Apart from the loud shots, there was the continuous humming of bullets flying past. We had to turn around in retreat, driving frantically back, with a number of students, caught up in the crossfire, clinging to our vehicle. Fortunately, 'Layi was, once more, able to fend off his attackers.

The next strike by NASU was once more about the Examination Administration Allowance. The members of the union downed tools on 6 October 2000. Initially, the municipal services were maintained, because the senior non-teaching staff was not on strike. The striking workers employed their usual tactics of violence and intimidation, particularly against academic staff, whom they increasingly considered as their enemies. They regarded them and ASUU as actively working against their welfare and progress. They attacked a number of members of academic staff, and, quite naturally, there were increasing calls from ASUU that its members should be protected from harm and the culprits brought to book. The attacks were becoming increasingly frequent and serious, and anarchy was gradually setting in. We identified a number of NASU members who were at the forefront of the violence. As before, Bimbo Awopileda was one of them. There was another man nicknamed "Artillery", a labourer in the Maintenance Department, who went about threatening violence to all and sundry whom he regarded as depriving him of his rightful earnings. He had attacked a number of individuals, and I actually witnessed him attack the Chief Nursing Officer, Mrs. Ogundana, in the Secretariat building. I had to rescue her. He also personally threatened me but did not actually lay a hand on me. Of course, they also employed and threatened with *juju*. A week into the strike, they surrounded the steps to my office with *raffia* rope, from which were hanging various charms. Arriving there, I broke through the obstacles and started to climb up the stairs. There were several NASU members picketing the area, and, as I went up, I heard one say, "I thought you said he would not be able to go up?" Another, presumably the *juju* man, answered, "Don't worry, he will not (be able to) come down." My subsequent descent and my apparent immunity to other incidences of *juju* attacks, presumably contributed to the widespread belief that I was immune from such preternatural agencies. On one occasion, the NASU Chairman, Niyi Akinnibi, told me that he knew I had a talisman!

When the situation was getting out of hand, I met with the Administration Team, and proposed to stop the salaries of the striking members of staff if the violence continued. I put out a release, which I personally signed, that was broadcast on the local radio and television stations. It outlined the events of recent weeks, and the escalating violence. It also stated that the strike had no justification and concluded with the statement, *"Aseju ti wo oro yi"* ("This matter has now gone to excess"). It ended with a statement that the salaries of the striking members of staff would be stopped with effect from the following Monday, 16 October, if the violence continued and if the striking members of staff did not return to work. I was later informed that this threat to stop salaries was received with absolute disbelief, indeed with hilarity. The union leaders told their members that they should not worry and that I would never dare stop salaries. Their response was to escalate the conflict by stopping the supply of water and power. On 13 October, they entered the water works and power house and switched off the power and the water supply, driving off the SSANU workers from the premises. They issued threats against any person who tried to restore the supply, and even made direct threats against those whom they had identified as being involved in such activities in the past. They went as far as visiting their wives and threatening untold horrors, usually involving the use of *juju*. When I went to see one of the electrical experts who had helped in the past, his wife refused to allow him to come out of the bedroom and had seized his clothes. I decided to go ahead and restore the two supplies on my own. Two nights later, I went into the power house through the fence at the rear, accompanied by some members of the Cracker Unit. I got into the power house and switched on the power. I then proceeded to the water works and operated the water supply system overnight. The only person who came to help was Wale Akinsola, but he had little knowledge of how to operate the systems and was able to provide only moral support.

In the morning, I left the water works and went back to the power house. While I was inside, NASU started holding a congress on the sports field. I locked myself inside the power house. I was determined that the power and water supply should stay on. An hour into the meeting, the NASU congress decided to invade the power house. Led by their chairman, Niyi Akinnibi, they broke down the gates and then started hammering on the doors of the building itself. I had requested Professor Adebayo to avoid getting the Police involved, but it was clear that my life was now in grave danger. I spoke to Wale Adebayo over a walkie-talkie and requested that the Police should come to my rescue. Soon after, the mob broke down the door and streamed in. The mob surrounded me and engaged in a protracted attack. I noticed that they were afraid, either of being identified or, as some subsequently asserted, of my personal power. Many of them believed I had a talisman that would protect me against them and also bring harm to anyone that came near. Because of this, rather than attack me directly, they would individually run in, beat me, and run back into the crowd. As with the Wesley Guild incident, they were armed with charms, including the notorious *"atori"*. Honestly, counting the number of times I have been flogged with *"atori,"* I should be dead by now or completely impotent! While the attack was going on, the mob switched off the power and started vandalising the equipment.

Things were getting hot. The mob was getting bolder and I

knew my life was in danger. However, I was not afraid. Rather, I had become more and more furious at the cowardly attacks. After some time, the blows subsided somewhat and Akinniyi came up to me and said, "Mr Vice-Chancellor, you have switched on the power. The next time you do so you will not survive it." At that moment there was a hubbub outside and in rushed a contingent of mobile policemen, headed by their Commander and the Area Commander, Mr. A.T. Shinaba. There was tear gas everywhere. The mob quickly dispersed, and the Area Commander told me to leave with him. I was very angry and initially stated that I was not going anywhere. The two commanders actually lifted me up bodily and carried me out.

The mob had caused major damage to the power house equipment. After the arrival of the mobile policemen, they also went to the water works and removed some of the fuses. The mobile policemen stayed on the campus for a month. It took us three days to restore the power and water supply. The Chief Technologist in the power house, Mr. Awe, managed to repair the damaged electrical equipment. I took Engineer Adams Ojo, a lecturer in the Electronic and Electrical Engineering department, to the water works and he was able to diagnose the problem, missing fuses, which my friend Prince Adewa supplied. Power and water supply were once more restored, and run by volunteers from the University community. Incidentally, we had to run the water supply with the aid of volunteers during a number of subsequent industrial actions. One of the most dedicated of these volunteers was Dr. Yemi Mojola, now a professor. She was an intrepid individual, respected throughout the community, dedicated to justice and truth.

At this time, the *Ooni* of Ife showed once more what a great source of support he was. He summoned me to the Palace for a briefing on the situation. After I explained things to him, he arranged for a meeting with the NASU leaders the following day. When I arrived, he sat me on a chair next to him, with his secretary kneeling between us. He then sent for the NASU leaders, who had been waiting outside the audience chamber. They came in and, as is the tradition, all prostrated. Kabiyesi did not allow them to get up. He asked, "Who is your leader?" From his position on the floor, Akinnibi raised his hand. Kabiyesi then said, "What do you want me to do after you have beaten up your Vice-Chancellor?" Akinnibi protested that they had not assaulted me. The *Ooni* said he knew they had. He advised them to return to work and find some accommodation with the University Administration. He dismissed them and they left.

I stopped the salaries of NASU members with effect from the date I had given, 16 October, which coincided with the day of the attack in the power house. They had not believed it was possible. It had never happened before in the history of the University. They confidently went to the bank to collect their salaries only to be told nothing had come in. The salaries were not paid for the remainder of the strike, which was called off on 17 November. Almost a year later, and following repeated pleas from the union and letters of apology for their behaviour, Council approved that the withheld salaries be paid. The Police rounded up three of the individuals who had been involved in the attacks and charged them to Court. They included Akinnibi, 'Lanre Awoyeye, and, of course, Bimbo Awopileda. "Artillery" managed to evade arrest. I found him later to be a reasonably pleasant character and a very hard worker. His actions were influenced by the psychology of the mob. Following the pleas and apologies by the union, Council also requested me to withdraw the cases against the three arrested individuals. The individual who struck the first blow in the power house was the storekeeper in the water works. After the strike was over, I saw him at work and reminded him of it. He became very agitated, and said, "It was not me. I was at the hospital with hypertension." I left him.

NASU had learnt its lesson. Its power was broken, and this time they knew it. Future industrial actions were not accompanied by violence and interference with municipal services. Indeed, the few industrial actions by NASU that occurred during the rest of my administration were fairly innocuous. SSANU had also learnt its lesson, albeit vicariously. Indeed, unless NASU joined them in a strike action, their powers were fairly limited. The Governing Council directed that the "No work, no pay" law be invoked for all strike actions, and it proved a very effective weapon. When SSANU embarked on a five-day "warning strike" in February, 2001, their pay was stopped for the period. It took several appeals and a letter of apology before Council agreed to release the withheld pay. The "No work, no pay" provision, combined with firm handling, proved effective with the non-academic staff unions, but, as we shall see later, it was relatively ineffective with ASUU.

The strike continued until mid-November, but at least we had water and power. Dr. Babalola, the Dean, Student Affairs, organised the clearing of the halls of residence. The University was closed for two weeks after the power house incident. As soon as we resumed, the postponed semester examinations were held successfully in spite of the strike. On a future occasion, we even held the examinations with both SSANU and NASU on strike. This further reduced the power of both unions—we had shown that we could successfully conduct this most important of functions without them.

We did have one more fairly prolonged strike involving both unions at the beginning of 2003. The two unions did rely heavily on their remaining weapon to ensure compliance by their members and to strike the fear of God into everyone else. By that time I was the "substantive" VC, and living in the VC's Lodge. I thought I had fairly loyal staff there, but the most senior of the stewards managed to convince the other two that the unions had invoked strong "medicine" and, if they valued their lives, they should stay away from the Lodge. Only Grace Odere, who had been working with my family since 1988, remained faithful. Fortunately, I had taken her along with me when I moved to the VC's Lodge and got her appointed on the staff of the VIP Guest Houses. She stayed with me, in spite of the threats against her. After that strike was over, I refused to have the stewards back. However, after a few months, Dorothy, while on one of her trips home, persuaded me to take them back. As usual, we were able to maintain municipal services through volunteers. By then, I was an expert on both the water works and the electricity system. So were several others.

One interesting episode occurred during that strike action. As I mentioned earlier, the two unions went all out to employ *juju*. I later learnt that during one of their congresses, they brought in a *Babalawo*. During the proceedings, the medicine man is said to have shouted, "Who is the VC? Show me his office" and made some incantations against me. I knew nothing about this, and, if I had, I would have laughed. I travelled to America on a study visit sponsored by the Carnegie Corporation soon after. However, during that trip I became progressively ill, with an intermittent fever. I had no appetite, was nauseous, and began to lose weight. I did not seek medical help in America because the Severe Acute Respiratory Syndrome (SARS) epidemic was at its height at that time; I was scared that I would be admitted straight into an isolation ward if I did. By the time I returned to Nigeria, I had a high fever and was deeply jaundiced. Those who saw me were shocked. Fortunately, Dr. Tony Akintomide, who, in my opinion, is one of the best physicians we have in Ife, sorted me out. I am sure the two unions believed that it was their *Babalawo*'s incantations that had gotten to me.

XIII

Governance

✦ ✦ ✦ ✦ ✦ ✦ ✦ ✦ ✦ ✦ ✦

While it is true that the period of my Acting Administration from July 1999 to May 2001 was overshadowed by the communal crisis and industrial problems, there were still some important developments. The Governing Council met in September and again in December 1999. During that last meeting of the year, we were about to wind up proceedings at the end of the first day when the Public Relations Officer, Mr. Afolabi, came in and whispered that he needed to speak with me outside. He told me that the Government had announced over the radio that it had dissolved all the Governing Councils of the universities. Apparently, this was in response to the reports of the visitation panels. I went back in and said nothing until the day's proceedings had ended. Having confirmed the story, I informed the Pro-Chancellor and then had to go from one member of Council to another informing them of the development. They had had no inkling that the Council was about to be dissolved and it was extremely embarrassing and distressing. They all departed quietly the following morning. This kind of dismissal over the radio used to be the practice of military regimes, and I had experienced it myself during the Buhari regime. However, I did not expect such insensitive behaviour from a civilian regime. Well, some wise people claimed the government of the day was only a military government disguised in civilian clothing! It was some months later before the Council members received "thank you" letters from the Ministry.

We operated without a Council for the next seven months while the Ministry of Education assumed responsibility for all matters for which Councils were normally responsible. This meant that I had to make frequent visits to Abuja. The Honourable Minister, Professor 'Tunde Adeniran, always received me with politeness and I found him to be a great help. Some weekends, he would invite me to his home in Ibadan when I had pressing matters for which I required his approval. He always approved any reasonable request that I put before him. He wanted the University to succeed, and had much sympathy for the troubles that we had been through. He had some innovative ideas about the university system, and he was the one who developed the original Autonomy Bill. I was shocked when he was unceremoniously removed from office in late 2000.

This was a time when funds were quite short. We were totally dependent on the Government for our funds. The recurrent subvention was barely enough to pay salaries. The Capital Grant had ceased, and was not restored until 2002. The only source of development funds was the Education Tax Fund. We had a total of 13 capital projects that had been abandoned at various stages of completion in the 1980s. We evaluated them and decided that the priority should be the completion of these projects. No new capital projects should be started unless an abandoned project could not be modified and completed to meet the particular purpose. The obvious exceptions here were, of course, student hostels. Indeed, most of the Education Tax Fund grant for 1999/2000 was allocated to the construction and equipping of four hostel blocks. The other major capital project that was ongoing was the Central Science Laboratory.

One important early development was the International School. The University had built a secondary school, Moremi

High School, on the campus in the late 1970s, which had been handed over to the then Oyo State Government. The school had developed into a first-class institution. The staff of the University was very happy with it. It was being run under the State's Free Education Scheme, with very high standards. Both of my children, Roger and Tony, attended the school. From the early 1990s, the school began to deteriorate. The standards declined, and this was aggravated by successive strikes by the teachers. The University, under pressure from the community, tried to get the school returned by the State Government, now Osun State, to the University, but this was resisted by the Ile-Ife community. Given the township's resistance, the Government considered it politically unwise to return the school to the University. One morning in October 1999, a delegation of the University staff came up to my office while we were having a meeting of the Management Committee and requested an urgent meeting. They complained that their children in Moremi High School had not been taught for over six months as a result of the on-going strike by teachers. They said, if the State Government would not hand back the school, then the University should establish its own private secondary school on the campus. We were ourselves very worried about the issue, which, after all, concerned staff welfare, and agreed that this was a valid option. I requested the group to come up with a proposal. I suggested that they should get the Dean of Education, Professor J.O. Fawole, involved as an adviser. They agreed and departed.

Two weeks later, the same six members of staff came back, accompanied by Professor Fawole. They were Dr. Yemisi Obilade, who later became Vice-Dean of Student Affairs, Dr. R.A. Togun, Mr. Tajudeen Ejalonibu, Dr. P.I. Oyeyemi, Dr. C.A. Makinde, and Mr. V.C. Ohalete. I asked for their report, expecting a comprehensive document with elaborate plans for the new school. Instead, Professor Fawole announced, "We have started the new school." They had actually gone out, identified temporary accommodation, recruited some teachers and enrolled students from among the children of the members of staff who were dissatisfied with Moremi High School. They had worked out the salaries to be paid to the temporary teachers and the fees to be charged. Three sites were to be used, and the owners of these sites had already released them. One was an unused block of the Government primary school on the campus, another was the unused block in the Staff Development Unit, and the third site was the laboratories in the Faculty of Education. Teaching had already commenced. I had asked for a plan, instead they presented me with a school. I discussed this *fait accompli* with my colleagues on the Management Committee and we agreed to support the school. We released some funds to help with the initial costs. The Committee continued with the development of the school, which was named *The OAU International School*.

We had a new school and now we had to get it approved. I tabled the matter before Congregation at the end of January 2000. Most members of Congregation were in favour of the new school. However, there were a number of detractors, who stated that we had acted illegally by establishing the school without first getting the approval of the appropriate university committees. I remember that the most vehement objections were raised by Dr. Idowu Awopetu, the then Chairman of ASUU. In my opinion, it was improper for him to give an opinion, since his wife was the proprietor of a private secondary school in the town. The meeting eventually agreed that the new school was necessary, and Congregation, after some discussion, gave its support. However, from the debate, it was obvious that we were going to face some problems.

The next step was to take the matter to the Development Committee. Here we were lucky. Professor P.O. Aina, the Dean of Agriculture, was chairman of the Finance Sub-committee, and he did some extensive homework on the financial and other requirements. The Development Committee gave its assent. The final stage was to take the matter to the University Senate. When Senate met on 2 February 2000, their reception of the proposed school was extremely hostile. This was a major development, yet no approval had been obtained before we had gone ahead. Speaker after speaker condemned what they saw as my nepotic actions in starting the school. I recall Professor Ogedengbe asserting, "This is a monumental breach of the University's procedures." Hardly anyone spoke in favour. Eventually, I asked, "Shall we cancel the school?" They shouted, "No"! They knew how important the school was to the University community, and they dared not stand in its way. Finally, the school was recommended for the approval of the Governing Council. That is how the OAU International School was established—by the determination of just a few parents and the Dean of Education. Over the next few years, we gradually developed the facilities of the school, and were able to withdraw from the initial temporary accommodation. We started with an interim Principal, Mrs. T.A. Oyebisi, seconded from the Registry, who got the school off to a good start, aided by the Interim Management Committee, some committed teachers, and a dynamic Parent/Teachers' Association (PTA). The first substantive Principal after Mrs. T.A. Oyebisi was not as successful as Mrs Oyebisi, but her successor, Mrs. A.O.L. Adeniyi, did extremely well. The school now has all the facilities of a first-rate secondary school, including hostel accommodation built by the PTA. I am very proud of the school.

***   ***   ****

My relationship with the ASUU leadership was rather dicey right from my assuming office. I guess they continued to be unhappy about the manner in which I had been appointed. I was also not regarded as one of "them" but as a person who went his own way. They were convinced that I would erode the Committee System which they held sacrosanct. The latter was not strictly true. I believe in the Committee System, which allowed all those with a concern in a matter to make their input and which also, at least in theory, militated against the nepotism that has so plagued our country, including the university system. However, I was also aware of its limitations, and made no pretence about these limitations. One morning towards the end of 1999, I arrived at the Minister's office to be told by his Special Assistant, Dr. Dipo Kolawole, "ASUU has written a petition against you." The Minister later asked Dr. Kolawole to show me the petition, which complained about my lack of regard for the laid-down procedures of the University, especially a disregard for what they called "Due Process." One of the major examples of this was the manner in which I had single-handedly "approved and implemented" the OAU International School. I later learnt that during a congress in which the main topic was the behaviour of the Acting VC, a committee had been set up to frame the petition on ASUU's behalf. The committee was chaired by Professor Jide Ige of the Department of Chemistry, who had already become a prominent source of opposition and criticism. The Minister told me not to worry about the petition but to get on with my work, and expressed his confidence in me.

At the end of June 2000, the Government announced the membership of the new Governing Councils. Professor Umaru Shehu, a very distinguished medical academic and experienced university administrator, was to be the new Chairman of Council. He had been Vice-Chancellor at Nsukka and sole Administrator at the University of Maiduguri, as well as Pro-Chancellor of two universities. I was delighted. I arranged to meet him and flew up to Maiduguri, where he was an emeritus professor in the university there. Professor Umaru Shehu informed me that, while he was delighted over his appointment, he would not be able to take up the post. He was also the Chairman of the National Programme on Immunisation and he had been informed by the Minister of Health that he would not be allowed to hold both positions and should decide which one to drop. He was committed to his work on the Immunisation Programme and had to decline the appointment as Pro-Chancellor. I left Maiduguri a very unhappy person. Sadly though, Professor Shehu was removed as Chairman of the National Programme on Immunisation a few months later.

I went back to the Minister, who told me he was looking for a suitable replacement. After about three weeks, I was informed that a suitable individual had been found in the person of Alhaji Shettima Liberty, also from Maiduguri. Alhaji Liberty was a lawyer. Throughout his tenure as Pro-Chancellor, I found him straightforward, honest, and committed to doing what he believed was right for the University. At that time, apart from the Pro-Chancellor/Chairman, the Governing Council had nine members appointed by the Government. They were supposed to represent community interests, but they were in fact mainly politicians, members of the ruling political party. There was also the President of the Alumni Association, the representative of the Honourable Minister of Education, four representatives of the University Senate, two representatives of Congregation, the VC, and the two Deputy VCs. The Registrar was Secretary to the Council. The Senate and Congregation representatives were all members of the academic staff. ASUU had a major interest in their election, and even decided who to put up and support. Some were so blatantly representatives of ASUU's interests that they used to go out in the middle of meetings to consult with ASUU leaders over the phone.

A few of the Council members stood out. There was Dr. (Mrs.) E.M. Irukwu, a retired teacher and author, who was a fountain of wisdom and also wielded a potent pacifying influence when things got hot. Professor B.I.C. Ijomah had been Registrar of a university and was also an academic. During the first meeting of the Governing Council, he insisted, repeatedly and very vociferously, that, in view of his experience of the university system, he must be on the Tenders Committee. The Pro-Chancellor diplomatically but firmly declined to place him on the Tenders Board. However, he was a very knowledgeable individual and usually gave valuable advice. Once when I insisted that Council should take a stand contrary to his advice, I came to regret it. Professor Mary Lar was the wife of the famous politician. She was also completely committed, decent and honest. Professor Idris Mohammed had been appointed Chairman of the National Programme on Immunisation after Professor Umaru Shehu. He had been Chief Medical Director of the teaching hospital at Maiduguri and was a highly respected academic. He had been my classmate in the University of Ibadan. He understood the important issues in the University. Mr. J.O. Ogunranti was a retired teacher, quiet, unassuming, but straightforward and honest. I got on very well with this very pleasant man. Chief Akin Omoboriowo is best known for contesting the Governorship of

Ondo State in the 1983 election. He won the election under very questionable circumstances but this was overturned in court. He initially gave me the impression of a man who wanted to contribute in his own way to the development of the University. He was very supportive. I spoke glowingly about him to my friends, who expressed scepticism and reminded me of his antecedents. I replied that, if he had been bad in the past, he had most certainly changed for the better.

Finally, I must mention Dele Oye, who was a very successful barrister in Abuja. He had been elected President of the National Alumni Association earlier that year. I was actually quite sceptical about him because of the manner of his election, which involved the mobilisation and transportation of masses of alumni to Ife from as far away as Abuja. This must have cost him a lot of money. He was even more sceptical about me. He had been informed by a member of the former administration that I was a highly dangerous person who was hell-bent on being made substantive VC and would go to any lengths to achieve this. He claimed that I employed *juju* widely, and, apart from occult means, was capable of sending assassins against him. He was in fear of his life on arrival and booked two rooms in the Conference Centre, one in his name, which he did not occupy, and a second in another name, in which he stayed! I believe it did not take him long to realise that I was a very different person from the one who had been described. I believe he soon understood that my only ambition was to succeed, and that, to me, success was simply that the University should develop into a first-class institution. We shared that ambition. He had a passion for his alma mater and he made enormous sacrifices for the University over the next four years. He also became a good friend.

The first meeting of the new Governing Council took place from 26 to 28 July 2000. NASU was on strike at that time, and, because of their violent behaviour, we proposed that the meeting should take place in the VC's Lodge. The Council members insisted that the meeting should take place in the normal venue, the University Hall. Among the important decisions taken were the ratification of the establishment of the OAU International School and the release of ₦15 million for the Staff Housing Loan Scheme. Following consideration of my report on the recent industrial crisis, Council endorsed the administration's actions and pronounced that the "No work, no pay" rule should be strictly enforced for any future strike action. The Council showed a genuine concern for the welfare of the university community and committed itself to the development of the institution. I was very pleased at the end of that meeting. I felt we had a Council we could work with.

XIV

A New Vice-Chancellor

At its second meeting in September, Council agreed to set in motion the procedure for the appointment of a new VC. It appointed Idris Mohammed to the Search Party. More importantly, it appointed Chief Omoboriowo and Mr. Ogunranti to the Joint Committee of Council and Senate that was to interview the applicants and recommend suitable candidates to Council. I was delighted about the two Council representatives. I had not known Mr. Ogunranti for long, but I regarded him as a very fair and honest individual. As I have stated earlier, I believed Chief Omoboriowo was also a decent, fair-minded person. He had been very supportive of me and frequently expressed the opinion that I was doing very well.

At its meeting of 27 September 2000, the Senate appointed its two members to the Search Party. However, the really important issue was the membership of the Joint Committee of Council and Senate. A number of individuals campaigned actively to be appointed. One of the candidates, Professor Bade Ajuwon, was heard stating that he was not going to contest for the Vice-Chancellorship on this occasion. He had contested in 1999 but now wanted to be appointed to the Joint Committee of Council and Senate, in other words, to be an *afi Oba je* (king maker). Professor Ajuwon and Professor Jide Ige were elected. This was the same Professor Ige who had chaired the committee that wrote the ASUU petition against me. I was not comfortable with this development.

When the Search Party arrived in my house, I informed the members that I had already submitted my application. As was their practice, ASUU organised a referendum, preceded by an interactive session with its congress. As I had done the first time round, I prepared a manifesto and circulated it on the University's intranet as well as in hard copy. I did not go around campaigning, as the majority of the other contestants did. However, I prepared hard for the interactive session with the ASUU congress, and I believe it went very well judging by the applause at the end of the session. I won the referendum by a landslide, a result that was not well received by the ASUU leadership, who once more refused to release the result to the media. By now, the result was popular knowledge. The ASUU leadership therefore had no choice but to write to the Governing Council listing me as the first choice of its members. The other unions also organised referenda, in which I was declared their first choice. Even the Students' Union organised a referendum, with the same result. These referenda have no legal standing in the choice of a VC; nevertheless, they do carry some weight, albeit unofficial. As with the 1999 exercise, various *juju* sacrifices started appearing around the campus, at crossroads and in the vicinity of the VC's Lodge. In addition, a number of the candidates began consulting with various Pentecostal Christian churches. I recall one candidate in particular who became as thin as a rake from protracted fasting.

My three referees were Professor Olikoye Ransome-Kuti, Dr. Tinuola Abiola-Oshodi, the former Chairman of the Hospital's Management Board, and Professor David Ijalaye, our long-time family friend and mentor. The interviews of candidates took place in the second week of February 2001. After presenting my proposals for the University, the rest of my session with the Joint Selection Committee was conducted by Professors Ajuwon and Ige. They requested me to explain various procedures and regulations, constantly referring to the University's Calendar and other handbooks which they referred to repeatedly. It was a ludicrous exercise, since, as I constantly reminded them, the answers were to be found in those books. At the end of the session, the Pro-Chancellor asked me if I had any questions. I replied that I had no questions but wished to state that Professor Ige had previously chaired a committee that had written a petition against me to the Government on behalf of ASUU, and was therefore unlikely to provide an unbiased judgment. Professor Ige responded, "Did I sign the petition?" I later learnt that the two Senate representatives had played a prominent role in the development of the scoring scheme. I will give only two illustrations of the bias that they brought into that scheme. My previous service as Chief Medical Director of the Teaching Hospital was given the same rating as headship of a university department. One of their favoured candidates had been the Dean of the Postgraduate School and was transformed into the Provost when the School became a College during his term. He was given ten marks for having been a Dean and another ten marks for having been a Provost!

The Joint Committee gave me a score of 53.2%, ninth out of the ten candidates. The highest score was 93.1%. The three candidates with the highest scores were then recommended to Council. Council considered the report of the committee on 20 February 2001. I withdrew from the meeting during the discussion, so what follows here is drawn from the minutes and what filtered back to me.

Many of the Council members were extremely critical of the exercise. They clearly thought the procedure had been flawed. The most prominent critics of the report were Dele Oye and Idris Mohammed. Arguments went back and forth. In the end, it was decided that members should be given further time to examine the report and that a special meeting would take place on 23 March to consider the matter further. I was also not present at that meeting. However, the minutes recorded that in recommending only three candidates to Council, the Joint Committee had usurped the duty of Council, which was to recommend three candidates. The Committee should have recommended more than three candidates and the number would then have been pruned down to three by Council. It was agreed that the report of the Joint Committee be accepted but not its recommendations, and that a secret ballot be carried out among Council members to decide on which candidates to recommend to the Government. I scored 10 marks, as did Professor Yinka Folayan. Professor R.O. Olaniyan scored 8 marks. Council decided to forward the three names to the Government in the following order – Makanjuola, Afolayan, and Olaniyan.

That was not the end of the story. At the next meeting of Council on 3 May, some internal members submitted a letter in which they tried to change the minutes of the previous meeting. After some angry discussion and a reprimand by the Chairman, the letter was withdrawn with apologies from the group. A period of intense lobbying followed. Some of the candidates spent more time in Abuja than in Ife. Religious consultations continued, and I thought one of the candidates would almost disappear—he had become even thinner after he resumed fasting. I did not go anywhere. However, I believe that my three referees interacted with those in power. I suspect that the *Ooni* may also have spoken to the Government on my behalf. If they did, I never asked any of them to do so. By then, Professor Babalola Borishade was the Minister of Education, and during the Opening Ceremony of the National Universities Games Association (NUGA), at which he was present, our University contingent shouted, "Roger, Roger, Roger!" I do not know if this influenced him or not.

Rumours were flying around. All three names were bandied about at various times as having been approved by the President. The visits to Abuja by the other candidates and their godfathers continued. One was said to have enrolled in the ruling party and had been guaranteed the job by a prominent politician who had the President's ear . I began to prepare my hand-over notes. On 7 May, one of the headlines of the 4 o'clock news stated, "New VCs have been appointed for Obafemi Awolowo University and the University of Jos." I was announced as the VC. I did not hear the news bulletin. It was the Registrar who first came into my office, and jubilating, told me about the appointment. The celebrations went on in my house until well after midnight. Dorothy joined in the celebrations over the phone. Uncle David Ijalaye, in his hotel room in Abuja celebrated with *suya* and heavy inroads into a bottle of Remy Martin. Aunty Joke represented them both in my house. We had a great time that night. The only drawback was that, having led a bachelor's existence for some years, there were only two drinking glasses in the house. My visitors had to make do with anything available, mainly mugs and teacups. No one complained at the time, but somebody must have reported me to Dorothy. When she received the reports of my uncivilised behaviour as a host, she expressed her displeasure in no uncertain way. She also made sure that, from that time on, whenever she came over, she bought loads of glasses!

XV

Strategic Planning

ⵡ ⵡ ⵡ ⵡ ⵡ ⵡ ⵡ ⵡ ⵡ ⵡ ⵡ

When you are in limbo, as I had been over the previous 22 months, it is difficult to make long-term plans with any seriousness. Armed with a five-year term, planning became essential. The university system in Nigeria was faced with major challenges. There was a major funding crisis, resulting from the nation's economic woes and the proliferation of universities that had been going on since the 1980s, and with which the declining economy could no longer easily cope. Misplaced priorities, corruption, and mismanagement present within all strata of the economy had, of course, exacerbated the situation. As with most Federal universities, the student population in Ife was at least four times larger than the teaching facilities and social services could accommodate. The grant for the payment of salaries was barely enough, and sometimes we had to rake funds together from other sources to pay salaries, especially when there was some addition to the wage bill such as the annual leave grant. The subvention for the running costs of the institution was ludicrous. At one point in 2001, the monthly running costs grant was ₦4.6 million. At that time, the monthly electricity bill alone was ₦7–10 million. Apart from funding, there was also the challenge of globalisation, with the Nigerian University System, which had been internationally isolated during the military years, now faced with the demands to achieve international standards and recognition. Allied to this was the challenge of harnessing modern technology, including Information and Communication Technology (ICT).

Universities are traditionally bastions of conservatism. Ife is no exception to this. In my opinion, the academic community in Ife is one of the most conservative in the world. Their response to proposals for change is usually, "This is not how we have done it in the past." Our community is highly resistant, and very slow to change in any area, whether it be supporting gender equity or adopting a less bureaucratic collegiate system, or in anything at all. By the way, I thought about trying to introduce a modern collegiate system but my feelers suggested a very hostile reaction to the concept. With regard to the funding crisis, it was clear that the University needed to diversify its sources of revenue and become less dependent on the Government. Such a proposal was anathema to the Ife community. The usual responses to any such proposal, by both academic staff and students were loud shouts of: "It is the Government's responsibility to fund education;" "The Government has enough money;" "If the Government stopped looting our economy, it would have enough funds," and other similar statements.

I put out proposals which were based on my manifesto. The aim was to achieve international standards and recognition for the University. We should not be comparing ourselves solely with other Nigerian universities, but aim to stand shoulder-to-shoulder with any other university in the world. These standards would apply not only to our degrees, research output, and impact on the nation and the local community, but also to the conditions under which we lived and worked. I presented comprehensive proposals for a progressive reduction in our dependence on Government funding. At that time, the Federal universities were not allowed to charge tuition fees, but I proposed a range of charges for the other services that we provided to students. Commercial activities and investments were also included, and, finally, there were proposals for international linkages and support from external funding agencies and donors. The latter were subsequently designed into the development of the Office of Linkages and Sponsored Research and the Advancement Office, about which more information will be provided later. The proposals also included a range of plans for harnessing modern technology, including ICT. These proposals were formally presented to the Governing Council, Senate and Congregation, and at meetings with the unions, including the Students' Union. Council appeared to receive them positively. The response from the other groups was lukewarm.

We regarded these as interim proposals which could be pursued while we developed a more comprehensive strategic plan. Strategic planning was currently receiving much attention from the Government, and the National Universities Commission put pressure on all the universities to develop their plans. We set up a committee to develop our Strategic Plan. I was officially the chairman, but Wale Akinsola was the de facto chairman and he spent a substantial part of the next two years on the job. I provided a lot of input in the Mission, Vision, and the seven broad Strategic Objectives, while the nitty gritty of the individual objectives and strategies were developed by the Committee, working with the various stakeholders. Strategic plans provide detailed proposals to cover a specific period, usually five years, as in our case. However, there are two unique concepts in strategic planning. First, it is participatory. All those who have a concern with the University are involved in its development—staff, students, the local community, the alumni, Government, you name it. These concerned parties are, of course, also those who are involved in implementing the Plan. Equally important, the Strategic Plan should contain realistic objectives and realistic strategies for achieving those objectives. "Realistic" implies that the objectives will be achievable. Based on the explanation above, developing a good Strategic Plan takes a substantial amount of time, resources, and effort. Ours took over two years before it was approved by Senate and the

Governing Council. The Mission, Vision, and the seven strategic objectives were as follows:

The mission of the University was to foster a teaching and learning community for imparting appropriate skills and knowledge, behaviour and attitudes, advance the frontiers of knowledge that are relevant to national and global development, engender a sense of selfless public service and promote and nurture African cultures and traditions.

The vision was to be of a top-rated university in Africa, ranked among the best in the world, whose products occupied leadership positions in the public and private sectors of the Nigerian and global economy, that had harnessed modern technology, social, economic and financial strategies, built strong partnerships and linkages within and outside Nigeria and whose research contributed a substantial proportion of innovations to the Nigerian economy.

The strategic objectives that were identified as critical to the achievement of this vision were:

1. To produce graduates of international standard, with appropriate knowledge and skills in their fields of study, who would be highly employable and also able to create their own employment.

2. To provide high quality research and development activities that would promote the development of the Nation and enhance the image of the University and its researchers.

3. To harness modern technology, especially Information and Communication Technology, and modern, social, economic, and financial strategies to run efficient and cost-effective academic programmes and institutional management.

4. To provide services that had relevance to and impact on the local community and the Nation.

5. To provide conditions of study, work, and living in the University community that were of appropriate standard.

6. To expand access to tertiary education in the face of unmet demand.

7. To operate as an equal opportunity educational institution, sensitive to the principle of gender equity and be non-discriminatory on the basis of race, ethnicity, religion or physical disability.

Following a statement of the strategic objectives, there were comprehensive specific objectives and strategies to achieve them. These were divided into five sections: Academic functions, Financial strategies, Administration, Staff and Student welfare, and the University estate.

I believe the Plan, which lapsed at the end of 2008, was a good one. However, it was obvious that some components were not realistic in terms of the financial resources required. We got on with it and we achieved many of the objectives by the time I left.

My family moved into the VC's Lodge on 5 July. This was a very special time for Dorothy and I. Apart from moving into this extremely beautiful building with its absolutely well-manicured grounds, our younger son, Tony, got married. To me the most important aspect of this event was that we were acquiring a daughter. We had wanted a daughter desperately in our younger days, but our wish had not been granted. We could not have wished for a more loving, truly good daughter than 'Wanne, Tony's wife. We now have two daughters, both acquired through marriage. Both are fantastic. God has been very kind to us in bringing Wanne, and three years later, Nicola, Roger's wife, into our family. Dorothy was home for the wedding, and so were Tony and his elder brother, Roger. A small group of friends joined us in the evening and Professor Adebona, whom we have known as neighbours since we arrived in Ife in 1978, said prayers. A week later we were in Benin City for the wedding, a spectacular affair. Wanne's parents, Justus and Bridget Nwaka, love their daughter as much as I do now, and organised a splendid traditional ceremony on the Friday and the church wedding on the Saturday. The event was covered by Ovation Magazine. We did not pay for that coverage. The proprietor of Ovation, Dele Momodu, is an alumnus, and I guess he authorised it. I personally drove the newly–weds from the reception to Ile-Ife in my Jeep.

Did I mention the Jeep earlier? I had a second-hand Toyota Camry which I drove to work and back and out of office hours. Dorothy felt that the vehicle was not befitting for a VC. One day in November 1999, during one of her trips home from Saudi Arabia, she told me she was going to Lagos to visit her mother. That evening I arrived home and saw a Mitsubishi Pajero in the driveway of our house. Dorothy proudly announced, "We have bought you a new car." She had gone with *Oga* Arigbabu and Mr. Layi Alabi and bought the Pajero in Lagos. I told Dorothy that I had not asked her for a new car and that I was happy with the clapped out Camry. Layi and *Oga* left in disgust. Dorothy was silent, but I could see she was furious. This is just one example of my tendency to assume a holier-than-thou attitude sometimes. I guess my reaction was because I was very sensitive to the university community seeing me in a new car. Actually, it was not a new car, it was 10 years old! Anyway, I soon came to my senses but was now faced with the problem of apologising to Layi and *Oga* and appeasing the wrath of my wife. It took some time. That Jeep proved invaluable. I drove it until I finally left the University in November 2009.

Anyway, back to the wedding. I drove Tony and Wanne from Benin to Ife. The following day we had a thanksgiving in All Souls' Church on the campus during the normal service and entertained a number of well-wishers in the Lodge. It was a grand occasion, but more importantly, a very happy one.

By now we were enjoying, with the exception of the ASUU leadership, a tremendous amount of goodwill in the university. The academic staff, particularly the younger ones, believed I was making a difference. The non-academic staff unions were still smarting from the manner in which we dealt with the strikes, but by the time the Governing Council approved the payment of their salaries, the majority of them had realised the excesses of their leadership. The students, with a few exceptions, were extremely supportive. They really believed that I was committed to their welfare.

XVI

Developing The University

As I have mentioned earlier, a major challenge facing the Nigerian University System was to develop facilities that would allow it to compete with other institutions in a global economy. For this, we needed the required physical facilities. However, equally important was to develop the capability of the staff to employ these facilities. Obviously, harnessing modern technology, including ICT, was one of the priorities. During Wale Omole's administration, the development of ICT had started, and the University was already leading the way in this field. It was decided that further development of ICT should be a major priority. The person who had been in the forefront of the ICT project, Professor G.O. Ajayi, had moved to Abuja as head of the national ICT development project soon after I arrived. I appointed his deputy, Professor Lawrence Kehinde, in his place. He performed brilliantly as Director of the Information Technology and Communication Unit (INTECU). Lawrence Kehinde is a very religious individual, a pastor, and a truly good person, but, above all, he is extremely capable. He later became the Deputy VC (Administration). Over the next seven years, Lawrence and his team developed our ICT facilities into the most advanced of any university in West Africa. The system is served by a Very Small Aperture Terminal (VSAT). We had begun with wireless connections to the local area networks. This was subsequently changed to optical fibre cable connections and "hot spot" wireless systems were introduced later. INTECU established a computer assembly plant that has produced Personal Computers for a number of institutions. We acquired the most advanced computer engineering laboratory in West Africa through a Carnegie Corporation of New York grant. One of the projects that has brought great credit to the University is the iLab project. This is a system of on-line practical experiments, whereby a student can conduct real-time experiments on-line from one centre using equipment in another centre. During a Carnegie Corporation sponsored US study tour for Vice-Chancellors in 2003, we were given a demonstration of the project at the Massachusetts Institute of Technology (MIT) in Boston. My immediate response was "You must bring this project to Ife." Subsequently, the Carnegie Corporation provided a grant for the joint development of the Project by MIT, the University, and two East African universities. We made great progress with this. Our students in the Physical Sciences were able to conduct sophisticated experiments on-line. We developed some experiments which were accessed by the other partner universities. Indeed, we were so far ahead in developing the system that the other two African universities were actually holding us back.

The academic and administrative functions of the University were progressively operated through ICT. Staff and students in the University have become increasingly dependent on this technology. Much of the finance for the development was provided by the Carnegie Corporation.

One other project that Wale Omole had started was the Central Science Laboratory. One of the major constraints to science-based research in Nigeria is the lack of functioning equipment. The Central Science Laboratory concept was to provide state-of-the-art facilities at a single site, available to all researchers in the University. I believed this system would be a major resource, and I was right. We gave full priority to the completion and further development of the Laboratory. The Laboratory was employed not only by our own staff; researchers came from universities all over Nigeria to use the equipment. The initial facilities included the only Nuclear Magnetic Resonance (NMR) Spectroscopy machine and the only scanning electron microscope in West Africa. There were a variety of other types of analytic equipment, all computerised. We later added a liquid nitrogen plant and facilities for Molecular Biology. Electricity was provided by two generators, one dedicated to the NMR equipment. All the equipment was stabilised and provided with an uninterrupted power supply back-up. Efficient management is critical to the success of such a system. As I mentioned earlier, Kwashi Ako-Nai, who also later became a Deputy VC, was in charge. He did a wonderful job in developing and running the facility, assisted by a dedicated team of academics and technical staff.

The Centre for Distance Learning was first proposed during my predecessor's time. The proposal was held up in Senate and the funds required for its development had also not been found. The proposal was eventually approved by the University Senate in March 2002. Council's approval followed soon afterwards. The Centre was to be responsible for all external programmes of the University, including our extremely successful and highly lucrative Executive MBA programme, as well as all our part-time programmes. New executive and part-time programmes were to be developed. I appointed Professor P.O. Aina as its Director. On his recommendation, I also appointed Dr. (now Professor) Rotimi Adagunodo as Deputy Director. Both applied themselves with great dedication and ability to the task of developing the Centre. By the time the Centre was approved, the buildings for it, to be provided by converting an abandoned power house project on Road 1, were not ready. They set up shop in a disused building within the academic area. Their first major development was the establishment of the Pre-degree Programme. This was a one-session programme providing admission to the University for those that passed the Programme's final examination. The

Programme started with borrowed facilities in a secondary school in Ipetumodu. Accommodation was organised in various homes in the town. Some landlords developed makeshift hostels for the students. This Programme was highly successful. It produced graduates that were better prepared, both academically and socially, for university life. Their products led the way in their classes in the University. The Programme also generated substantial funds, which were shared by the Centre and the University. The Centre's share was used for the development of facilities in Ipetumodu. There, a rapidly developing campus was established, both for the Pre-degree and other programmes. This story would not be complete without a mention of Professor M.S. Akanni, the same individual who was so angry with me at a Senate meeting. He was the first Coordinator of the Programme and applied himself to the task as though nothing else mattered. The success of the Programme was largely a result of his efforts. We used to call him "Mr. Pre-degree." Earlier, he had applied himself as Head of the Chemistry Department with the same degree of ability and commitment. A truly remarkable man.

The physical development of the University is guided by a Master Plan, developed in the early life of the University. Successive administrations have followed this Master Plan, and we stuck firmly to it. As I mentioned earlier, the campus was littered with abandoned projects that had been started in the 1980s and then abandoned when the economic problems of the country worsened dramatically. We decided that priority should be given to completing these projects. New projects would be approved only if one of the abandoned projects could not be adapted for the purpose. This applied to the Central Science Laboratory, which needed a purpose-built building, and student hostels, which had to be sited in the area designated for the purpose.

The first project we completed was the building for the Institute of Cultural Studies, much to the delight of our former Vice-Chancellor, Professor Wande Abimbola. He had proposed this to establish a niche for himself in the Institute. It is a great pity that he never did return to work in the University after he vacated office. I was the eighth VC in the history of the University. Four did not complete their terms. Of the remaining four, I am the only one, so far, who returned to work in the University after his term ended.

The building for the Institute of Agricultural Research and Training is an example of a project that was adapted to a different purpose. We completed one of the blocks for the Faculty of Environmental Design and Management, which had been established 20 years earlier in temporary accommodation. The abandoned power house project on the main university road was adapted and completed for the new Centre for Distance Learning and the Central Technology Laboratory Workshop.

The construction of student hostels was a major priority. Between 1999 and 2004, we completed ten hostel blocks, including three for clinical medical students, who had previously been poorly provided for. One of the most important major projects was a link road between the University and the Teaching Hospital. This has greatly facilitated the work of the medical school and provided easy access to members of staff needing hospital care. A number of lives have been saved in emergencies. If that road had been constructed earlier, Seni Osunade, the medical student murdered during the communal crisis, would probably have been alive today.

Much of the capital expenditure went on the rehabilitation of facilities. The Ife campus was regarded as one of the most beautiful in Africa. The students and alumni boast that it is the most beautiful. This beauty is based on both its architecture and its horticulture. Over the years, both had deteriorated. The natural environment still remained beautiful, though less so than in its earlier days. However, the buildings had suffered considerably. Most of these beautiful buildings had been constructed in the 1960s and early 1970s. Most had not received even a lick of paint since then and the infrastructures had also severely deteriorated. This deterioration had been greatly made worse by leakage from their flat roofs. We were determined to return these buildings to their original beauty. The first priority was to repair the roofs, and initially, much of the rehabilitation funds went into this.

We repaired the majority of roofs of major buildings on the campus over a five-year period. The University's Renovation Project, which restored the beauty of a large proportion of the major buildings towards the end of my term, will be dealt with later.

Funds were short, and we had to be prudent in awarding contracts. There was no room for major contractors like Solel Boneh or Costain. We had to employ smaller, indigenous companies, but we tried to make up for that with good supervision. Solel Boneh, one of the biggest civil engineering contractors in the country at the time, had started the abandoned University Hall extension. We wanted the company to complete the project, but their bid was almost twice our own estimate. We had to give the job to a more competitive but less known contractor. Fortunately, the contractor, Basilica Builders, did the work well, though far behind schedule. The project was actually completed after I left office.

With one or two exceptions, we had a great team working on our capital and rehabilitation projects. Bayo Amole, an architect who has been a close friend since the mid eighties, was the Chairman of the Projects Advisory Committee of Council when I assumed office. Soon after I arrived, the Chairman of the Projects Implementation Committee resigned. I appointed Bayo in his place. I reasoned that the functions of the two committees were related, and the two would be best integrated, and I was right. The system worked extremely well. Bayo is a gifted and committed professional. Through these two committees, he organised and supervised the projects very efficiently. He was much respected by the technical staff. The Director of the Physical Projects and Development Unit, Wale Ayodeji, a highly competent engineer, was also completely committed., We had a good team. We got our projects completed to a high standard and in a most cost-effective manner. We worked to a high standard of integrity, though there were some exceptions. The contractors responded to our expectations. They knew we were honest. They did not have to do anything underhand to win contracts. They also knew they would be paid promptly for any work they did, provided it was to the correct standard. Actually, I used to type the payment approvals myself. I had a number of templates on my computer which I would run off as necessary, usually within 24 hours of the receipt of the payment certificates. I did not approve any payment unless I had seen the work myself. We used to go round regularly as a team to inspect projects and interact with contractors, so we were always abreast of the progress of each contract. If necessary, I would make a flying visit with the Director or Bayo before approving a payment.

Most of the members of staff were honest, but there were some exceptions. One of the projects executed with the special grant from the Government to combat the secret cult menace was a fence around Mozambique Hall. During an inspection visit, I found I could easily look over the fence. Since the fence was supposed to be two metres high and my height was 1.92 metres, I queried the payment certificate on the project that I had received the previous day and which had been certified by the Quantity Surveyor on the team. I refused to approve the payment. The Quantity Surveyor was issued with a query. Also, when his papers for promotion came to the Administrative Staff Committee, I vetoed the promotion. On another occasion, we discovered that another quantity surveyor was part of a company that had secured a contract to build a student hostel block, and had actually been involved in the construction work. She had to go, much to my regret, because she was a rather competent professional. Integrity had to come first over any other consideration.

One of my biggest mistakes in office was the appointment of a senior officer in the Works and Maintenance Services. In the early period of my appointment, he was active in the Alumni Association. I was infected by his enthusiasm for his alma mater, and also by his apparent honesty. Also, I had developed the conviction that the University's alumni were all sincerely committed and they would never fail the institution. How wrong could I be in this case? I went out of my way to recruit him. At first, all my expectations were met. He showed great enthusiasm and dedication. He gave the impression of an action man, much in line with my own approach. As an alumnus of the University, I wholeheartedly trusted him. Gradually, I came to realise that he had very limited professional competence, which he covered up by his talk and enthusiasm. A year into his job, a contractor approached me, complaining that the senior officer had been demanding and obtaining money before he would issue certificates. I did not believe him, but when he agreed to put the complaint in writing, I set up a Panel to investigate the allegation. The Panel cleared him. However, I continued to receive complaints and information about his extortion of money from other contractors. I made personal enquiries and received very disturbing reports about his integrity. I felt let down because, in my opinion, the university's alumni could do no wrong, particularly in matters relating to their alma matter. He was one of only two alumni who disappointed me during my seven years as VC.

Apart from the renovation of our buildings and infrastructures, two major rehabilitation projects made an immense impact. The Teaching and Research Farm, once the pride of the University, had progressively declined during the 1980s and 1990s. One of the reasons, of course, was shortage of funds. Another reason was the failure of those involved in its management to adapt to the changing financial situation. From the start, the farm was run purely as an academic facility, with no major attention to income. Money was ploughed in, and, although some income was generated from the sale of produce or services, little regard was given to balancing income against expenditure. You could buy almost anything there, including fresh milk, but nobody was counting the cost. This was all very well when money was plentiful, though how you could teach agricultural economics in such a situation beats me. When funds did become scarce, most of the Faculty just folded their arms. The farm progressively deteriorated into a moribund desert. In the mid-1990s, some efforts were made to resuscitate poultry farming, but these had limited success. Towards the end of 1999, I had a discussion with the Dean of Agriculture, Professor Funso Sonaiya, on the possibility of resuscitating the farm and operating it on a more sound economic basis. The challenge I put to the Dean was for the farm to generate enough income at least to sustain itself and also its continued development. We agreed that if he produced a viable proposal, I would seek the Council's approval for the required funds to resuscitate the farm. Once that initial fund was provided, no further grants would be requested or given.

I took the proposal to the Council in September 2000. Council expressed support for the project but requested further business analysis. A grant of N11.1 million was finally approved a year later. However, nothing happened for the next three years. A tractor with implements had been ordered, and two successive Deans took no further steps, stating that they were awaiting the arrival of the tractor. Even after the tractor arrived, it sat idle in the Secretariat car park for a year.

When Professor Sina Aderibigbe became the Dean of Agriculture in August 2003, he immediately set to work, and personally supervised the development and running of the farm. The poultry business was revived and expanded. He repaired the feed mill, much to the annoyance of local feed mill ventures in town, which could not compete with the prices and quality that the farm provided. Extensive crop planting was done, mainly of maize and cassava. Most of the other areas of activity were revived. At last, the farm looked like a farm, with a good range of crops, a noisy and highly productive poultry, a piggery, and even the beginnings of cattle farming. The oil palm plantation was cleared and a substantial quantity of palm oil was harvested on a yearly basis. The farm started generating income during Sina Aderibigbe's time, meeting Council's objectives. It provided not only its running costs but also funds for its continued development. The Dean had a group of excellent individuals working with him, but it was his leadership and his example that really drove it to success. Even at weekends, Sina would be on the farm, sometimes driving the tractor. In addition to the new tractor, he repaired the two broken-down tractors that had been condemned some years before. The story of the farm is a great example of what can be achieved by capable and determined people. I regret that after he left the Deanship in 2005, the development of the farm lost momentum. However, on my most recent visit in 2010, I was delighted to see that things were moving once more.

The University's land is very extensive. Most of it has not been developed, and is home to a large variety of trees, which add greatly to the uniqueness and beauty of the environment. During the 1980s, the university set up a sawmill as a commercial venture. This was done without regard for the conservation of our beautiful environment. Profit was the order of the day. Even though the University was felling and selling its own trees, the sawmill ran at a loss and soon closed down. One theory for its closure was that most of the really valuable trees found their way to other sawmills in the town and not to that of the University. However, the real tragedy was the enormous damage done to the environment. Wide swathes of the University's rain forest had been cut down. The view from the hills was of devastation. This problem was compounded over the years by the activities of poachers, who appeared to operate without hindrance.

Early in 2000, I was approached by Dr. J.O. Faluyi of the Department of Botany with a proposal for a reforestation of the campus. The project involved extensive tree planting of economic trees, including oil palms and teak, which would then be managed conservatively. A tree nursery would also be set up. Thus, after a take-off grant was provided, the project would be self-sustaining. I took the proposal to the Governing Council, which approved a grant of N3.4 million in September, 2000. The project, which involved a team from the Department of Botany headed by Dr. Faluyi, achieved extensive planting of trees on the University's land. The tree nursery was particularly successful, and generated great profit from sales. They even supplied seedlings to as far away as Abuja. As one drives or walks through the University's land, one is struck by the evidence of the efforts of Dr. Faluyi and his dedicated team.

XVII

Student Affairs

¤ ¤ ¤ ¤ ¤ ¤ ¤ ¤ ¤ ¤ ¤

Over the course of my tenure, many reports in the media concerning the University related to issues with the students, mainly crises. Indeed, much of my time was engaged in dealing with the students and their problems. The crises were a feature, but most of these dealings were positive. As will be seen, I had an extremely turbulent relationship with the student leaders. However, I sensed that, even during the periods of greatest confrontation, the majority of the students truly liked and respected me. We had an excellent team in the Dean and Vice-Dean of Student Affairs, *Bablo* and Yemisi Obilade. I must mention another valuable individual in the Student Affairs Division—Mr. R.G. Oduola. He truly understood the students, had great compassion for them, and was a great negotiator during crises. My approach was markedly different from that of my predecessors in that I was easily accessible. I have been criticised for this. Many members of staff, particularly the more conservative, believed that the Vice-Chancellor should be dignified and distant, and that, if he was too easily accessible, he would lose the respect of the community. These same individuals never complained if I was too accessible to them. To be a distant deity was not my style. I felt that these were young people who had been traumatised by the 10 July incident and who had lost confidence in the University Administration. I did not think it unbefitting to visit the halls of residence regularly, sometimes in the company of the Dean, and sometimes on my own. I usually drove there in my personal car. Risky, you might say, but most of the time I was well received. When there were problems in the halls, I would be there. I tried to show that I cared, and I did care. It wasn't mere show. When the new students came into residence, I would go to their hostels (mainly Angola and Mozambique Halls, which were designated for new students) in the evenings to find out how they were doing. Many of them were as young as 15 or 16 years and were very vulnerable. One night when there was a serious fire in Akintola Hall, I got there to find the place in a state of pandemonium. The students, all females, were shouting and screaming in terror. Electricity had been cut off, so there was total darkness. I calmed things down and got the Hall Leaders to sort out accommodation for those whose rooms had been burnt. Calm was restored. The Hall Chairman and the students were full of gratitude, and as I was leaving, the Hall Chairman said "Sir, thank you for caring".

I also showed no fear, at least externally. Soon after I arrived, I was told that the Students' Union President, Lanre Adeleke, had made a false statement about me. I cannot remember exactly what it was. I drove to Awolowo Hall and confronted him in front of a group of students. He withdrew the allegation. The Hall Chairman then invited me to join in their *Ewa* (beans) Day celebration. I did and ate a plate of beans that had been prepared in a communal pot.

I tried to promote interaction between the Students' Union and the Administration. This had limited success because of the hostility of most of the union executives I worked with or, should I say, tried to work with. Students are represented on a number of university committees, and I encouraged them to attend these meetings. The most important was the Advisory Committee on Student Affairs. The previous Administration, apparently in response to the repeated student crises it had experienced, had removed them from membership of that body. I got Council to put the students back on the Committee.

The halls of residence were in a sorry state. They were terribly overcrowded. The official allocation of bed spaces meant that the spaces between beds, which were mainly bunk beds, were just about wide enough for someone to stand up. This officially induced overcrowding was made worse by "squatting"—an arrangement whereby other students would live in the rooms, often sleeping on the floor.

The University has its own water supply system, but its output was inadequate. Thus the halls of residence suffered from chronic shortages of water. If there was a breakdown in the system, even for a few hours, the situation became intolerable. There was another factor which made the situation even worse— the attitudes and behaviour of the students. The students, both male and female, appeared to have no regard for cleanliness and sanitation. They deliberately littered their surroundings. In Awolowo and Fajuyi halls, they would throw refuse down from their rooms onto the ground outside. Once, when I confronted one of the students after I caught him doing this, he replied, "some people are paid to pick it up." On several occasions, I saw students dropping peel from food items to the ground, even when there was a waste bin next to where they were standing. In Mozambique Hall, the girls indulged in what they called "shot put." Because the toilets were in such bad condition, they would defaecate into a plastic bag and throw it into the surrounding bush. These practices were rampant. And yet I am certain that the majority of the students came from good homes. When I asked if they would treat their own homes in the same way, the answer was always "No." The culture of the halls was responsible. These young people arrived in the halls as decent girls and boys but were soon changed by exposure to a culture of filth and irresponsibility.

We made hostel construction a priority, and built ten hostel blocks between 1999 and 2005. We also worked to develop the "Student Village," a site just outside the campus set aside for private hostel development. The first privately owned hostel, contracted by UNIFECS, the institution's consultancy agency, was completed in 2000. A number of others followed, including a large two-storey hostel built by Ambassador Gunju Adesakin. The alumni also completed three hostel blocks for female students, including the 56-bedspace Alumni Hall. However, these additional hostels did not make a significant difference to the problem; the numbers were just too staggering. A private hostel development scheme sponsored by the Federal Government was established, but nothing came of it. The financial institutions involved in providing loans to the prospective contractors took a substantial amount from each of them as a "deposit" but never came up with the loans.

The expansion of the water treatment system was beyond the University's resources. We negotiated a Federal Government grant for a project to expand the system by 50% through the then Minister of State for Water Resources, Prince Awotorebo, an Ife indigene, who was well disposed to the University. However, the funds were never released, presumably because the Minister fell out of favour and was replaced. We carried out some maintenance work on the system, so that the plant was kept running at full capacity. In this respect, Professor Gabriel Makanjuola (not a blood relative), was indispensable. Professor Makanjuola is a highly respected academic and the inventor of many items of equipment, including the prototype mechanical yam pounder which was copied by the Japanese. He is one of the few academics who are also very proficient in the practical aspects of their profession. He was a real hands-on man and could solve any practical problem. He repaired many of the components of the water treatment plant, and even constructed some replacements. His approach verged on the obsession, such that given a task, he would abandon everything else and work on it until it was completed. I once arrived in his house with a pressing problem on a Sunday morning as he was about to go to church. There and then, he abandoned his family, leaving them to go off to church without him, and proceeded to the water works. His family saw no more of him until late evening when he drove home having put our "backwash" system back into order.

Through the efforts of a bright young engineer, Kayode Adeloye, the water supply system to the hostels was improved using a number of innovative schemes. These included the expansion of the pipeline network, diversions of supply to particular areas on rotation and resuscitation of gravity storage. Incidentally, the introduction of periodic diversions of water supply also helped to provide water to some areas of the staff quarters that had previously received no water. In Angola, Mozambique, and the Postgraduate halls, deep wells also provided an additional supply. Two boreholes donated by the State Government failed. We later discovered that the drilling team had diverted some of the screening and casing materials to their private use, so that the boreholes were useless.

The Dean, his deputy, some of the hall masters and I put major effort into encouraging the students to take more responsibility for their environment. I found that success was very much dependent on the leadership of each hall, particularily the Hall Chairman and the Hall Master or Mistress. I remember in particular that Mozambique Hall, occupied mainly by new female students, was greatly improved by the efforts of the three successive Hall Chairmen and Dr. Durosinmi, the Hall Mistress. They brooked no nonsense and also led by example. "Shot putting" ceased, and the residents began to take pride in the cleanliness of their hall. Sadly, this was not the case with Fajuyi Hall and Awolowo Hall throughout my seven–year stint. They remained the most unnsanitary of the hostels. On one occasion I spent my own money engaging cleaners to clear the accumulated filth that had been deposited outside each of the blocks in Fajuyi Hall, thrown down onto the ground over a period of weeks. I challenged the students to maintain the environment afterwards. A clean environment was restored for a short time, but within two weeks, the filth had accumulated once more. In 2005, I organised a competition for the cleanest hall. Mozambique Hall was the clear winner, followed by Angola Hall, the hostel for new male students. Fajuyi Hall was second to the last, and Awolowo Hall remained far away the last.

We made hostel maintenance a priority, and I believe this did make a difference. We increased the number of maintenance staff serving the halls, and also allocated more funds for the supplies required. These funds were generated from the introduction of the hostel maintenance charge. I personally supervised the annual repairs and renovation exercise. Here, once more, it was demonstrated that determined students and hostel administrations could work wonders. In the earlier years, the students were not particularly involved. Actually, they were not keen. They presumably felt that such activities were the responsibility of the University Administration. In 2005, following my training in a strategic leadership course at Johns Hopkins University, I held a meeting with the executives of all the halls, their Hall Masters, Fellows and Wardens, and the Division of Student Affairs. My new expertise included a root cause analysis technique for identifying the factors involved in a problem and the level at which they operated. During the meeting, I also emphasised participation in projects by the users. We held a protracted discussion to identify the problems of maintenance of the halls and their environments. At the end of this, we put together a proposal that would decentralise the repairs and place the responsibility on the Hall Management Committees comprising the student executives, Hall Masters, Wardens and Fellows. The Student Union leaders who participated in the meeting rejected the proposal. The Hall Management teams adopted the idea enthusiastically. We went ahead. Based on submissions from each team, we released the required funds. The work was never done better, and never done so economically. The staff of the Works and Maintenance Services division were very unhappy about having the job taken away from them. They must have felt greatly embarrassed about non-professionals doing their job and doing it so well.

I was much closer and more accessible to the students than most VCs, with the possible exception of Professor Oluwasanmi, the second Vice-Chancellor of the University, who sacrificed so much while building the University. During my walks around the halls, I was generally treated with great respect by the students. There were occasional distant shouts and boos by some Awolowo Hall students. I was unmoved and felt perfectly safe most of the time. The times when I experienced unpleasantness were when the Students' Union leadership was engaged in any of its confrontations. Even when there was no crisis, some of the student leaders would go out of their way to be confrontational and rude to me. They wanted to present a macho image to their fellow students and forgot what the university was about. For example during one long vacation, I was going round inspecting some renovation work in Awolowo Hall, when I came across a student in a block that was being re-painted. Since students should not have been occupying rooms in the block under renovation, I asked the student what he was doing there. He continued sitting on his bed and told me it was none of my business. He then harangued me for two or three minutes about the incompetence of my administration. I later found out he was the Chairman of the Hall, nicknamed Olembe. Everyone with me was shocked, but I held my peace. He was one of those I had suspended following a subsequent riot. Another young man, Isiaka Adegbile, who had been suspended from the University five years before but had refused to vacate the halls, confronted me aggressively on a number of occasions.

I believe that most of the students were of good character and held me in high regard. The student leadership often did not. I had no problems with the Executive led by Lanre Adeleke ("Legacy"). We worked extremely well together and had a very trusting relationship. I thought quite highly of him, and even attended his wedding after he left the University. I am not claiming that he was a saint, indeed some of his actions in the past deserved to be condemned. He was by and large an excellent leader, and I particularly admired the manner in which he restored order and security among the students in the chaotic aftermath of the murders. However, the "interrogations" in the Awolowo Hall "coffee room" which resulted in the deaths of two young people was sheer brutality.

My difficulties with Union executives started with the executive led by Adeniyi Akanni Adenekan, nicknamed "Dr.

3 As." I have been told that his hostility towards me started from the day of his inauguration on 18 February 2000, when I gave a speech praising the leadership of his predecessor, Lanre Adeleke (Legacy), and asking the new President to live up to his example. I also joked that he should wait until he passed his final examinations before he could call himself "Dr." He belonged to a militant political group called the "Pacesetters," which was in competition with the "Democratic Socialist Movement" (DSM or "SCAP") to which Legacy belonged. There were a number of other student political movements, but the Pacesetters and DSM were the most prominent. Adenekan criticised me at every opportunity, and had the tendency to turn any event into an opportunity for abuse. On one occasion, when the main transformer caught fire, I personally rushed to the scene. After the fire had been put out and repairs commenced, he led a group of students to the scene. Rather than ask how they could help, he made a speech stating that the fire was a further example of the Administration's failure to maintain the University's facilities. In March 2001, he claimed to have found a hand-gun in a hall of residence. He issued releases and held a student congress, claiming that the halls were under threat of a secret cult attack. The students were terrified. However, he repeatedly refused to hand over the "gun." After a week of increasing tension on the campus, he handed it over. It was a toy! He was a sneaky character who would provoke or order an action and then hide in the background while his colleagues took the action and exposed themselves to the heat.

During his time as President, he organised a number of violent protests. During these protests, vehicles would be hijacked, the university roads and gates would be barricaded and members of staff would be abused and assaulted. On one occasion, he led students to Osogbo to protest over electricity shortages and members of the NEPA staff were assaulted and some of their vehicles hijacked. The group was arrested by the police, but Adenekan, who always stayed in the background, escaped. I had to speak to the Commissioner of Police and request the release of the students with the condition that I would ensure that they were disciplined. I also apologised to NEPA over the disgraceful incident. In another episode during 2000, he and three others were sent before a disciplinary panel following a violent demonstration; I forget what the demonstration was about. One of them, contrite, immediately requested a pardon, which I granted. A second appeared before the panel, which recommended that he write a letter of apology. He complied, received a warning and got pardoned . Adenekan and the other student repeatedly refused to appear before the panel. This was his pattern of behaviour throughout my time as VC. One of the major issues was the demand for the reinstatement of a group of student leaders called "The Ife Eleven" who had been suspended in 1995 after a series of reprehensible actions that had culminated in the disruption of the University's Convocation Ceremony. This was a truly disgraceful episode. Nevertheless, I was in support of their reinstatement in the belief that after six years they had suffered enough punishment and that you should never give up on a young person. A more important reason was that this would promote peace in the University.

Adenekan led a number of violent demonstrations in support of reinstatement. All they achieved was to alienate the University staff further. I repeatedly advised a more peaceful approach, but Adenekan did not see reason. The turning point came in September 2000, when Adenekan was impeached by the Students' Union and suspended for six months. The Vice-President, a very principled lady named Subumi Iginla, took over as Acting President. She raised the matter with me and I arranged for her executive to meet with the Pro-Chancellor, Alhaji Shettima Liberty. He expressed sympathy for the case, and advised them, as I had earlier, to adopt peaceful means to secure their objective. Soon after that, she informed me that the Union was insisting on a demonstration in support of reinstatement. I advised her to ensure that it was peaceful. It was, and I believe that this achieved a more sympathetic ear from the University community. A resolution of the matter was finally promoted by the visit of a Committee set up by the President in mid-2001 to assist in resolving the problem as well as in some other universities that were faced with the same problem. The Committee, chaired by Chief S.K. Babalola, an Ekiti politician and confidant of the President, was inappropriately named the "Resolution Committee on Politically Victimised and Rusticated Students." In the case of the "Ife Eleven," they had not been politically victimised, they deserved their punishment. Nevertheless, the Committee's activities were certainly influential in the reinstatement of the students. However, the efforts of Subumi also influenced the outcome. The Governing Council expressed support for their reinstatement and referred the matter to the University Senate. Senate was initially reluctant, and the matter went back and forth between Senate and Council. Eventually, Senate gave its reluctant support and the Governing Council pardoned the eleven individuals in 2002.

My decision to reinstate the eleven students, and my support of it, will always be controversial. The students had behaved abominably, and their expulsion from the University was fully justified. However, they had suffered severely. They were reinstated only after seven years. Nevertheless, there were resentful murmurs and criticism of me that we were sending out wrong signals to the students by reinstating them. On balance, I do not regret the reinstatement of the eleven students. All of them came back to the campus and applied themselves to their studies. They also set an example through their good behaviour. Nine of them subsequently obtained their degrees. One left without a degree, but is now a successful entrepreneur. The last, a medical student and former President of the Union, graduated as a medical doctor in 2010. You should give young people a chance, and they can make success of it.

At this point, one of the most truly horrific event involving the students will be described. The names of those involved and the date of the occurrence are being withheld for legal reasons. One night, a young man was apprehended near the Students' Union building. He was caught in possession of large quantities of cannabis, and was obviously a drug dealer. He was taken to the Awolowo Hall "coffee room," and, over a two-hour period, was subjected to a protracted and brutal beating with the claim that he was member of a secret cult. The brutality included beating him with planks supervised by some of the Students' Union officers. Among those who administered the beating were a Students' Union officer and an executive member of the Hall. The brutality ended when the young man was losing consciousness. He was then bundled into a vehicle and taken to the Security Post in the University Hall and handed over. On arrival, he was observed to be gasping and was taken to the Health Centre where he was pronounced dead on arrival. Wale Adebayo woke me up with the news. We proceeded to Awolowo Hall where the students who had been known to be participants in the brutality denied knowledge of it. We reported the matter to the Police, who invited the perpetrators to the Area Command Headquarters for interrogation. None of them went, and the Police were afraid to come to the hall because, a few years before, a Police Officer had been almost lynched when he went to arrest a student there. This young man who died was an Indian hemp trader and thus a criminal. There was no evidence that he was a secret cult member. Even if he was, did he deserve to be murdered? I am ashamed to admit that this gruesome incident happened when I was in charge and yet the perpetrators of this vile act were able to get away with it.

Adenekan's reign ended on a rather sour note when he was suspended for part of his term. However, as will be seen, he continued to feature negatively on the sidelines of activities of the Students' Union. Next came Yinka Sotade, nicknamed "Burkina Faso." He did not belong to any political group, but appeared to have enjoyed the support of the DSM. He was a student of Microbiology, but did not like the course, and eventually transferred to the Faculty of Education to major in Psychology. From the start, he stated that he wanted peace in the University and would work with the Administration to promote the welfare of students and the image and standards of the University. He was true to his word, to the annoyance of some political groups with a tradition of confrontation with the University. This militant faction considered him to be too cooperative and not confrontational enough. Even the DSM turned against him.

However, during his one year in office, things were peaceful and we were able to work with his Executive to promote student welfare. When a team from the Carnegie Corporation of New York visited the University in 2002, they met with Burkina's Executive and were quite impressed. Burkina's Executive did make a positive contribution to the eventual decision by the Carnegie Corporation to support the University. Unfortunately, as a result of his lack of militancy, the Students' Union congress suspended Burkina after nine months. His suspension was preceded by an extremely unstable one-month period during which there was much in-fighting within the Union, as various groups fought for control of the leadership. Threats to life were the order of the day, and there were a number of serious assaults. At one point, when she considered that Burkina's life was in danger, Juliet Dixon brought him to the VC's Lodge in the dead of the night. He was clearly shaken by what he had gone through. I had to lodge him in a room in the VIP Guest Houses for several days, while a group of students were actively searching to deal with him.

Next came Akinkunmi Olawoyin, nicknamed "Revolution." Right from the word go, he was confrontational. During his inaugural address, he announced that he would fight it out with the University Administration, though he did not say what the fight would be about. The tradition at such ceremonies was that the new President should bring up his executive, introduce them to the VC and I would shake each of them by the hand, encourage them to work with us and be of good behavior and wish them well. He ignored this tradition. Towards the end of the ceremony, there was a power outage. He announced that he would proceed to the power house and force the staff there to restore the power. I left immediately for the power house and was there when he arrived with a group of shouting supporters. They broke through the gate of the compound and rushed up to the building. They met me at the door of the power house and he demanded the immediate restoration of electricity supply to the halls of residence. I informed him that we ran the generators on a roster, and that we would be sticking to it. He and his group started shouting angrily and threatened to invade the power house. Just then the NEPA supply came back on. I then informed him that, as a result of his actions, electricity supply would not be restored to the halls for another hour. Olawoyin was nonplussed. He knew I would not budge, and he needed to save face in front of the students. He and his followers stayed outside the power house, singing militant songs until the hour was up, when I ordered supply to be restored. They then returned to the halls shouting that they had forced me to restore supply.

In spite of this discouraging beginning, we tried to work with Olawoyin's executive. We got nowhere. He appeared to be more interested in confrontation than constructive activity. Rudeness was the order of the day, and in this respect, only his Public Relations Officer, Ekundayo Fadugba, could rival him. Nothing we did had any value. Even when we were engaged in projects to improve the conditions in the hostels, he and his colleagues would look on. He was a member of the Pacemakers, and Adenekan was always in the background during his many forays into non-constructive criticism and, often violent, demonstrations. After the shooting of a student outside the supermarket in the Staff Quarters, the supermarket run by the wife of a senior member of the academic staff, was shut down for some time. After wide consultations over months and a religious service outside the premises, the supermarket re-opened. Soon afterwards, Olawoyin led a band of students to the premises and attempted to break in. They marched to the nearby Staff Club looking for the proprietor. Fortunately, she had left. They then confronted the President of the Club and two of them, whom we identified, attacked him, one holding him from behind while the other slapped him. I felt that the threats to the wife of a member of staff and the physical assault on a member of the academic staff were serious matters. I therefore set up a panel to investigate the matter in compliance with the University laws. In spite of the seriousness of the incident, the ASUU Executive conspired to get the students involved let off. Indeed, the sittings of the panel were disrupted by a group of academic staff led by their Chairman, Dr. Otas Ukponmwan, under the pretext that

ASUU was on strike and that the members of academic staff on the panel were not allowed to participate in such activities.

Olawoyin and his executive started to protest over the investigation, and also against the disciplinary actions taken against some other students. On one occasion, in response to a breakdown of the University's power supply which also affected the water supply, the students called a congress and invited me to address it. I went. After my arrival at the venue, Olawoyin addressed the congress, rudely criticizing how I had handled the problem. He then invited Adenekan to address the Congress. Adenekan continued with the abusive criticism and introduced the issue of some of the suspended students, demanding their immediate reinstatement. When I rose to address them, I explained the situation about the power and water supply and the actions we were taking. In fact, by then, electricity had been restored and pumping of water had commenced. I was about to leave when the students demanded that I address them on the issue of the students who were facing disciplinary action. My response was that the disciplinary actions would take their course in accordance with the University's laws and regulations. The next thing I knew, the gates were locked, and Olawoyin announced, "The gates are locked. The VC cannot go until he has agreed to reinstate them and stop the disciplinary panels." I went to the microphone and announced, "You have made a mistake by locking us in (the Dean of Student Affairs, some other members of his office and some other academic staff were also in the amphitheatre). You have made a mistake. Their suspension will continue." Olawoyin appeared crestfallen. After another 15 minutes the gates were opened and we left.

Olawoyin even took his fight with me to Lagos. In October 2002, a series of public meetings were organised by the Government on a proposed autonomy bill for the universities. We were invited to make a representation at one of the meetings in Lagos. I was not in the country at the time, and the Deputy VC (Academic) led our delegation to present a paper developed by the University Senate on the matter. Olawoyin organised a noisy demonstration at the venue, raining abuses on my person and claiming that I had embezzled the ₦15 million grant that the Government had provided to combat cultism after the 10 July murders. The Deputy VC and other members of the delegation were harassed by the demonstrators whose behaviour was a disgrace to the University.

The student leaders were always on the look-out for excuses to cause trouble. The power house was a frequent focus of protest, because of the fairly frequent power outages from NEPA and our limited power generating facility. The members of staff there were understandably concerned, and I had given them an assurance that I would ensure their protection. On the night of 5 July 2003, I was informed over the walkie-talkie system that a large group of students had invaded the power house and kidnapped a member of the staff, Mr. J. Odumade. I drove to the scene, to find an angry mob of about 100 students milling about. Mr. Odumade had been bundled into a commercial vehicle and was about to be driven off to Awolowo Hall. I had to get into the vehicle with him to prevent this from happening. The driver was terrified and so was Mr. Odumade. The bus was otherwise full of students who insisted that the kidnapped individual be taken to Awolowo Hall. Oddly enough, none of the known student leaders was around. The most vociferous of the band was a tall, dark-complexioned young man identified as Kunle. I suspect he was not a student, because he did not make any attempt to hide his identity. Kunle insisted that Mr. Odumade must be taken to Awolowo Hall and that I must come with him. He thoroughly abused me, and at one stage stated, "Let us naked him and carry him." Professor Adebayo, the Librarian, and the Dean of Student Affairs arrived on the scene, but no one could control the mob. While various individuals kept running in, kicking me and then running back into the crowd, I continued to insist that Mr. Odumade would not be taken away. I promised that I would personally come to the Hall 30 minutes later and address them. In the end they agreed, released the hostage and dispersed. I drove to Awolowo Hall 30 minutes later, entered the cafeteria where a large group of students had gathered, and mounted a table. They had, presumably, expected a long speech and discussion. This is what I said: "This evening, an innocent member of staff was kidnapped. Also, I have been attacked and kicked. There is a price to be paid." I then walked out, to loud protests. I got into my car, a heavy Pajero jeep, and drove off. I did not get far. They had laid a barrier of poles and stones across the driveway. I was immediately surrounded by a mob, shouting that I must come back and address them. I refused. The mob increased in size, shouting and banging on the car. This went on for over 30 minutes. At one point they lifted my jeep back a distance of about 50 metres. By then, Wale Adebayo, the Dean of Student Affairs, and the Librarian were on the scene, but were helpless. The whole area was dark, and I knew I was in real danger. Suddenly, the mob disappeared, running for their lives. The Dean of Student Affairs cleared the barrier and I drove off, followed by the others. To this day, I do not know what led to the dispersal of the mob. It was said that someone shouted, "Cracker n'bo!" ("The Crackers are coming"), but I have not come across anyone who actually heard those words. I believe it was a miracle. I believe there was a plan to cause me serious harm, to kidnap me or even to kill me. Those who planned it knew of my commitment to protect the power house staff; I had always come to the scene whenever they were under threat, and they knew I would come to the scene on that occasion. They took the opportunity of the power failure to quickly organise the invasion and my subsequent detention.

A more serious event occurred a few months later, at the beginning of the 2002/2003 session. The University had been finding it difficult to maintain the halls of residence. In 1998, modest charges had been approved. However, when they were implemented at the beginning of the 1998/1999 session, there were violent protests by the students, and the surcharges had to be temporarily withdrawn. However, the problem remained. The funds required to run the halls, the electricity and water supply, the cost of cleaning, and so on, as well as repairs and renovation, were just not there. Council had shelved the matter, but it remained on its books with a view to re-introducing the charges at an appropriate time. During the last sitting of the

Aniagolu Council in December 1999, the Administration was asked to review the proposed charges and advise on a suitable time for their introduction. At a special meeting on 22 June 2000, Senate decided that the charges should be re-introduced. However, with the arrival of Alhaji Shettima Liberty's Council, the matter had again been put off, quite reasonably, in view of the recent tragedy in July 1999 and the need to ensure peace in the institution. Eventually, revised charges were taken before the Governing Council in July 2001 and approved for implementation. The charges were ₦2500 per bed space per session, along with a Sports Levy of ₦1000. We informed the Students' Union of our proposal. They would have none of it. We decided to go ahead. We had to, if we wanted to provide decent standards in the hostels. We advertised the new charges both on the campus and in the newspapers. We also informed the Students' Union of the charges at a meeting. Naturally, they objected. Just before the resumption of the 2002/2003 session, we received information that the Union planned to disrupt resumption over their opposition to the new charges. We met with the Executive once more and they continued to express their opposition to the charges.

At the beginning of each session, new students normally come into residence first, followed by the "stale" students a week later. We had advertised the new charges in the newspapers. The fresh students came into residence on 26 May 2003. They and their parents happily paid up. However, during that first week, Olawoyin and his cronies organised a series of violent demonstrations. They rampaged through the campus, violently disrupting the collection of the charges and the registration of the fresh students. The new students were scared stiff. A Dean and some senior administrative staff were physically assaulted. Registration documents were seized and destroyed. On the second day, they padlocked the gates leading to some faculties. The padlocks had to be cut off by a member of the Works Division whom I summoned for the purpose. Isiaka Adegbile, the suspended student who had refused to leave the campus, was particularly violent. In the Faculty of Administration, he violently confronted the Dean, Professor Ojo, who called me to come to his rescue. When I arrived at the scene, Adegbile was storming through the lecture theatre where registration was taking place, throwing the heavy furniture around. He was like a mad dog. The Dean of Student Affairs with me and some others had to go round, confronting the rioters and at the same time reassuring the fresh students and their parents. Apart from Adegbile, Olawoyin and Fadugba were equally disruptive. On one occasion, Olawoyin and a group of his cronies surrounded me clapping and shouting abuse while Olawoyin danced around me. We stood firm. The fresh students all paid up. I consulted with the Legal Officer, and was advised that if a student committed an offence in my presence, then there was no requirement for an investigation. I suspended those who had committed acts of serious disrespect and/or violence in my presence for one session each. These were Olawoyin, Fadugba, Hassan Abass, and Olugbenga Adewale—the same person who had been rude to me in the Awolowo Hall Annex a year or so earlier. While their suspensions did not stop them from continuing with their misbehavior, as will be seen, it did dampen the enthusiasm of their followers. Incidentally, as was usually the case in such situations, the rioters were not all students of the University. They included young people recruited from the town and students from other universities. One student from the University of Ibadan, Stephen Tolulope Alayande, was particularly prominent. He even confronted me and identified himself. I wrote to the VC of his university, but received no reply. We could not do anything about Isiaka Adegbile, beyond reporting him to the Police, because he had been rusticated some years before. He continued to be harboured in Awolowo Hall by the students. He had caused trouble before, and he would cause trouble again.

On the second day of the protest, they hijacked a bus, led a mob to the town and collected a large number of old tyres. We received information that the tyres were to be set alight the following day and employed as barricades. I had already informed the security agencies of the possibility of trouble.

At the end of that second day, I requested the Police to come into the campus. A contingent of Mobile Policemen arrived the following day and stationed themselves outside the Library. However, the rioters by-passed them at the beginning of each day and continued to harass the staff, the new students, and their parents. On one occasion, at the entrance of the Faculty of Agriculture, a group of students seized a State Security Service officer and were making off with him. I had to rush to his rescue. The kidnappers ran off when they saw me. Wale Adebayo subsequently told me that they were afraid of being suspended following the suspension of their leaders.They knew that I had the power to take such action against students who committed offences in my presence.

We had expected that when the remaining students came into residence, there would be even more trouble. Happily, the protests abated, most likely because of the police presence as well as the knowledge that I had the powers of summary punishment for offences committed in my presence. The students all paid, with the exception of those who were genuinely unable to and who we exempted from paying. The Division of Student Affairs had a very effective system of identifying such individuals, as we were committed to ensuring that no student was deprived of education in OAU just because they were poor.

The suspensions provoked a worldwide reaction. The students wrote to other student groups as well as human rights organisations all over the world, and there were a number of publications in the hardline left-wing international press. I received emails from all over the world, condemning the action of the University in suspending the student leaders "for fighting for their rights" and condemning me as a fascist. I developed a reply, stating the facts and providing the rationale for the charges as well as a breakdown of the charges, which amounted to about US$25 annually. I actually got back one reply which apologised and stated that they were now better informed. There was even a letter from the Honourable Minister of Education, to which I replied along the same lines. I suspended the four student leaders on 26 May. In less than one week, their lawyers had gone to court, seeking permission to enter a case for the defence of their fundamental human rights and obtaining an injunction against the suspensions. I had no choice but to obey the order of the Federal High Court. They were reinstated and Olawaoyin and Fadugba continued in their roles in the Students' Union Executive.

These are just examples of the confrontational acts of Olawoyin and his Executive. His term ended after a year, but that was not the last we heard of him. He continued to feature in most of the future confrontations between the student leaders and the University Administration, as did Adenekan, the last but one President.

Next came Mohammed Elegbede, nicknamed "MM," who was elected in February 2004. He was probably not a member of any particular political group, but had been on the periphery of the student leadership for some time, and was to be seen hanging around the Students' Union offices. I had first come across him a year earlier, after he led a group of students to Trinity Tops Tutors on the Ede Road, a remedial school for those seeking entrance to university. A student had reported at the Students' Union that he was prevented by the Principal from entering the school to see a female friend. Elegebede led a group of students to the school and harassed the Principal and students. The Principal reported the matter to me. I investigated the matter along with the Dean of Student Affairs. Although the students in the school had clearly identified Elegbede as having been the ringleader, we could not pin him down because of a cover-up by his accomplices. I was apprehensive about his appointment because of this previous event. Although he was militant, he was not so much of a problem as his Public Relations Officer, Peter Olowokandi. The difficult relationship continued. By the time the "Ife 11" had been reinstated, there was now agitation for the withdrawal of punishment meted out to the four students involved in the May 2003 episode, as well as the cases against those involved in the assault on the President of the Staff Club. All the cases were in court. The Administration's position was that the cases in court should be concluded and that we would abide by the decisions of the court. Alternatively, they could withdraw their cases from the court and make an appeal to the Governing Council, which might be inclined towards clemency if the students showed adequate remorse. Neither of these options was acceptable—the Union leadership embarked on confrontation, and used every opportunity to press its case, employing threats and abuse.

The financial problems of the University continued. The National Universities Commission had persuaded the Government to introduce a new Direct Teaching and Laboratory Costs grant in addition to the recurrent subvention. This made a difference, but was nowhere near enough to support the costs of the delivery of lectures and conduct of practicals. The response of many departments was to introduce unofficial charges on the students, a practice which was unlawful and also open to abuse; indeed, it was abused. It was clear that, if the University's academic standards were to be sustained, charges would have to be introduced to support teaching. Following discussions at all levels, Senate proposed a number of charges to students, the most important of which were Departmental Teaching Charges and a Library levy. The Departmental Charges were to be employed for the provision of the equipment, materials, and other resources required for teaching. The highest of these charges was to be ₦20,000 per year for medical students in their clinical training years and Pharmacy students from their second year onwards; the lowest was for students of the Humanities, who were to pay ₦5,000. The Library levy was to be ₦1,000 per year. The new charges were approved by the Governing Council in April 2004. The charges were advertised and a number of meetings were held with the Students' Union Executive on the matter. Needless to say, the students strongly objected and vowed to resist the new charges. The Administration was extremely worried about the threat of violent disruption. Just before the resumption for the 2003/2004 session, scheduled for 25 August 2004, we met with the Executive and proposed an interim payment of 50% of the proposed charges. The Governing Council would then be requested to confirm a reduction of the charges to 50%. That decision was taken by the Administration. We did not have a Governing Council at the time and there was not enough time to take the matter to the Senate. However, we considered it expedient in order to forestall a violent crisis of major proportions. We planned to seek ratification of our actions subsequently. The Students' Union Executive expressed its acceptance of the reduced charges. We heard nothing further, and advertised the reduced charges.

We were hopeful that, with the reduction of the charges and the apparent agreement of the Students' Union Executive, a crisis would be averted. We were wrong. Fresh students came into residence on 25 August. A group of about 50 students went on the rampage immediately. The Students' Union President, "MM" was apparently not involved. I did not see him and received no reports of his participation. Rather, the protest was led by Peter Olowokandi, the Public Relations Officer, with the prominent participation of a student named "Taiye." The students rampaged through the academic area and halls of residence, threatening and physically assaulting members of staff, the fresh students, and their parents. Once more, these young people, proud of their success in getting into "Great Ife" had to repeatedly flee in terror. A number of them were injured. On their rampages, the mob confronted and abused anyone in authority. As with the year before, I with the Dean of Student Affairs, some other deans, and the Chairman of the Security Committee, had to go round, trying to restore order and reassuring the fresh students and their parents. On the third day after resumption, I came across "Taiye" and Olowokandi in the Faculty of Education. "Taiye" confronted me, pointing at me from a foot away shouting, "You are a thief! You are a rogue!" I immediately suspended Olowokandi for two sessions. Taiye could not be immediately identified. Following a tip-off that he was a Part III student of the Department of Dramatic Arts, I went to that Department and asked to see the files of the students in the class and so was able to recognise him as Taiwo Hassan. His identify was further confirmed by other members of staff who had been initially reluctant to reveal it. I suspended

Taiwo Hassan for two sessions. Both went to court, confident that, like their predecessors, they would obtain an injunction against the University and be reinstated, pending the outcome of the substantive case. This time, the court did not grant their request for lifting the suspensions. However, the two refused to abide by their punishments. Olowokandi declared that he was still the Public Relations Officer of the Union, and continued to wreak havoc. I requested for a contingent of Mobile Policemen to maintain peace. They arrived on the campus on 30 August. The "stale" students came into residence on 6 September. On 7 September, the students held a congress. Immediately afterwards, they invaded the Secretariat building, driving away the security men and ascending to my office on the fourth floor. Their spokesman was Olowokandi who made the following demands:

- The recently introduced charges should be scrapped.
- The two students suspended the previous week should be reinstated, along with those previously suspended or who were facing disciplinary actions.
- The accounts relating to the charges that had been introduced the previous year should be presented to them.
- The University Administration should address the Students' Union Congress that day.

I firmly refused the demands. However, I did state that the Administration was prepared to meet with their Executive, provided that no suspended student be present at such a meeting. I also informed them that the audited accounts of the University would be made available to them. The mob left, but invaded my office again later in the afternoon. They barricaded the University Hall so that no one could leave. After two hours, the Mobile Police, who were stationed at the Library, close to the University Hall, moved in and dispersed them with tear gas. Fortunately, there were no serious injuries to students, staff, or policemen. The disruption continued with less force afterwards, but we were able to complete the registration of the students. All of them paid the new charges, except, as in the previous year, those who were exempt.

The University Senate met on 8 September and approved our actions. It also directed that the academic session continue as planned. Lectures resumed, and for a while, things were peaceful, although there were still meetings of small groups of students during which the agitation for the cancellation of the new charges and the reinstatement of the student leaders continued to be voiced. Olowokandi and Taiwo Hassan, protected by their colleagues, refused to abide by their suspensions and remained on campus. Olowokandi even led a mob to the power house on 17 October during a power cut.

On Thursday, 21 October 2004, an interview was conducted for the appointment of a new Principal for the University's International School. Dr. D.F. Burgess, the Principal of Olashore International School, was our external assessor. As the interviews proceeded, we heard a commotion outside the room. It was a student demonstration. After a few minutes, the demonstrators moved away. I contacted the Security Department and was told the demonstration had ended and the students had dispersed. Half an hour later, the commotion was repeated and a group of about 30 young people, students as well as non-students, burst into the room. Peter Olowokandi, Taiwo Hassan, and Adenekan, the former Students' Union President, were among them. Their spokesman was Olawoyin, the former President who had earlier been suspended but reinstated following a court order. He made three demands—the reinstatement of those student leaders who had been suspended or were facing disciplinary actions, the release of the results being withheld by ASUU, and welfare issues, which particularly concerned electricity and water supply. However, it was obvious that the real issue was the demand for the reinstatement of the two student leaders who had behaved so disgracefully. I reassured the members of the interview panel of their safety and then addressed the mob. I informed them that the suspensions and other disciplinary proceedings would stay. The request for reinstatement of the two suspended students was a matter for the Governing Council. I stated that some of those present were guests of the University and that they should be treated with consideration and respect. I then requested them to leave. The response was that no one would leave until their demands were met. Once more, I assured everyone of their safety. Dr. Burgess stood on a table and addressed the mob, stating that he was only there to help the University. The students insisted that they must stay. The Dean, Student Affairs, arrived and spoke with the students. Still, they were adamant. I continued to insist that the disciplinary proceedings and punishments would stay. The student leaders then went into discussions with the Dean. After some time, Olawoyin announced that the Administration had agreed to reinstate the suspended students and drop all other disciplinary proceedings. I immediately stated that this was not true and that the punishments would stay. I was looking at Taiwo Hassan at that moment and I saw his face fall. After another hour, Dr. Burgess and the other guest were allowed to leave. We stayed on. Eventually, five hours after they had burst into the room, the mob left.

I issued a release the next day describing the incident and affirming that: "The two students will serve the full terms of their suspensions. Their reinstatement is out of the question. A clear message must be sent to the effect that students cannot perpetrate acts of gross misconduct and get away with it. Also, it would be against the interests of discipline, peace, and security in the University for punishments to be reversed through acts of violence and intimidation. We must restore decency to our community."

The crisis rumbled on, with the students holding congresses at which they repeated their demands. Olowokandi and Hassan were still in the forefront. One Thursday in October, I returned from running my clinic in Ilesa to find that a large group of students had once more invaded the Secretariat building and ascended to my office. Not having found me there, they were milling about on the stairs and on my floor. I went up the stairs through the protesters and entered my office, which a mob had occupied. They were too surprised to do anything except gape. They left. The militancy by the Students' Union was escalating.

I felt it was important to keep the university community fully informed, and drafted a lengthy explanation of the University's position on all the grievances which was released by the Registrar.

On Monday, 1 November 2004, the students organized a rally at the Sports Centre. Peter Olowokandi signed the invitations to the rally. The Staff Unions were invited and representatives of ASUU and SSANU participated in the rally. The ASUU representatives included Dr. H.C. Illoh, the ASUU Chairman, Dr. Otas Ukponmwan, Professor Idowu Awopetu, and Dr. Chijioke Uwasomba. The security report stated that Dr. Abiola, the ASUU Branch Secretary, was also present but I later discovered that he was not there. The Chairman of SSANU, Mr. Tajudeen Ejalonibu was also present. The rally was presided over by Olowokandi. It centred on the students' grievances and demands, which included:

- Reinstatement of suspended students and the dropping of outstanding disciplinary actions against student leaders.
- Release of the results of the 2002/2003 Rain Semester examinations.
- Welfare issues, particularly the conditions in the halls of residence and lecture rooms.
- The removal of the Vice-Chancellor.

The rally decided that a two-day lecture boycott should take place on 3–4 November, and that it should be accompanied by a total disruption of the functions of the University. It was also stated that kidnappings would take place during the period. The Staff Union representatives gave their full support to the decisions of the students. The Chairman of SSANU, Mr. Ejalonibu, went further to declare that the VC must be removed and that he would personally participate in driving him from his office during the planned disruption. In the event, he did not actually participate in the subsequent violence. Following the episode of hostage taking on 21 October 2004, the Dean, Student Affairs Division, met with some Students' Union leaders and gave an undertaking to facilitate a meeting between the students' lawyers and the University Administration. This meeting was arranged for Tuesday, 2 November. However, an hour before the proposed meeting, we were informed that the lawyers could not come on that day. Nevertheless, we met with the Students' Union Executive for about two hours. The President of the Union was not present, and their chief spokesman at the meeting was Mr. Kekemeke, the Speaker. There was a full discussion of the demands of the students. The students did insist that the lecture boycott would go ahead. They were advised to ensure that the laws of the nation and the regulations of the University were respected and that the rights of others were not infringed upon during the proposed action. Our readings of the mood of the students suggested that they would certainly be violent.

After the meeting with the students, Wale Adebayo and I discussed the matter with Mr. Shinaba, the Area Police Commander. I wrote to the Commissioner of Police to inform him of the impending crisis and requested that the Police should be in readiness to come to the institution's assistance if this became necessary. The Area Commander promised to have a contingent of Mobile Police ready to come into the campus. I had been planning to travel to Lagos for the Annual General and Scientific Meeting of the West African College of Physicians the next day. The meeting was particularly important for me, because I was campaigning for election to the post of President-Elect of the College, which was to take place during the meeting. However, I postponed the trip with a view to seeing out the planned demonstrations. That night, a white Nissan "Danfo" bus, Registration Number AH827EGD, was brought into campus and parked overnight outside the Postgraduate Hall. This bus was to play a major part in the proceedings of the following day.

The next day, Wednesday, 3 November, groups of students and non-students barricaded the gates and other key sites from about 7am. I went to my office as usual shortly after 7am. The Deputy VC (Academic), Biodun Adediran, arrived in his office at around 8am, and later joined me in my office. At about 8.30, I was informed over the radio that a mob of about 500 students had formed and was proceeding from the halls of residence towards the academic area. Soon afterwards, the mob arrived at the "Motion Ground," the area in front of the Library, between the University Hall and Oduduwa Hall. Peter Olowokandi and some others then insisted that they should invade the VC's Office and bring him down to address them. The majority refused, including most of the Students' Union officers. However, Olowokandi led a group of 50 to 100 individuals into the Secretariat building and they stormed up to my office. They shouted and banged on the doors and windows for about 10 minutes, and then burst in, with Olowokandi at their head. Among them was Adenekan, the former President, Isiaka Adegbile, and Olawoyin. They were shouting and screaming abuse. Peter Olowokandi, the suspended student, led them into the office. They damaged property and spread dirt and rubbish all over the room. Olowokandi stated, "The VC must come and address us. If he refuses, we shall carry him." The mob then subjected both Biodun and I to a protracted physical assault and insults.

Three members of the Students' Union executive came up to the office some time after the entrance of Olowokandi and his mob. Apparently, they had received information that things were getting out of hand and had come up to try and to restore sanity. These were the Vice-President, Caroline Akinsowon, the Secretary-General, Abiodun Ogundele, and the Speaker, Mr. Ojupiragba Kekemeke. They initially joined in the demand that the VC should come and address their congress. However, when the mob started to assault the two of us and began damaging property, they tried hard to restrain them. Incidentally, the President, Elegbede, was nowhere to be seen during the entire period. He subsequently claimed he had travelled out of the campus some days before the incident, and did not return until some days afterwards! The mob actually turned on the three executive members, and I had to restrain the Vice-President from fighting them. Olowokandi's group far outnumbered the few Students' Union officials who had come up to calm the situation. Faced by my continued refusal to come down, they left the office briefly, consulted, and rushed back in again. I was then carried bodily out of the room and into the corridor. Biodun asked me to give him my glasses as I was being bundled away. At first, I thought I was going to be hurled over the corridor wall to my death seven floors below. However, they carried me along the corridor to the stairs. I struggled hard, and repeatedly grabbed hold of whatever handholds I could find. Each time, they pulled my hands off from these. A member of the Bursary staff, A.O. Oketunde, was shouting to the mob *"E gbe"* ("Carry him"). I was carried down to the ground floor and onto the "Motion Ground."

I was continually kicked and beaten. I was repeatedly floored, and would struggle to get up only to be beaten to the ground again. A student nicknamed "Old Soldier" was particularly brutal, and was observed to repeatedly kick me, even when I was on the ground. He was identified as 'Muyiwa Aderibigbe. The assault lasted an hour or more. I was surrounded by a mob of about 50 people. Some wore handkerchiefs tied around the lower parts of their faces. I presume these were our students who feared recognition. Those students without masks faced me without any apparent fear of recognition, and I presumed that these were not our students. I was later informed that those who planned the incident had recruited students from the polytechnic in town as well as the polytechnic at Iree, and that some were members of a secret cult. Eventually, I was dragged across to the front of the "Motion Ground,", where a bus, the one parked overnight outside the Postgraduate Hall was waiting. Adenekan was inside the vehicle. The mob shouted out that I should get into the bus, which was to take me to Awolowo Hall. I refused, and continued struggling. About this time, the Dean, Student Affairs, Dr. Babalola, arrived, followed shortly afterwards by Professor Joseph Fabayo, the Dean of Social Sciences. They were also battered, and someone picked Professor Fabayo's pocket. By this time, my watch and both my cell phones had also been stolen. Both *Bablo* and Professor Fabayo tried to persuade me to enter the vehicle, so that the battering would cease. I said repeatedly, "I am not going anywhere." However, eventually I agreed to go and was about to enter the bus when a contingent of Mobile Policemen arrived, led by the Area Commander, Assistant Commissioner Shinaba, and accompanied by Wale Adebayo. The Mobile Policemen were armed, but initially employed tear gas.

As soon as we were rescued, there was a confrontation between the students and the Police. More tear gas was fired, and there were gunshots. I was terrified that some of the young people might be shot, and both Professor Adebayo and I pleaded frantically with Mr. Shinaba that nobody should be shot. He reassured us, stating that they were only firing into the air. The students were eventually driven back to the halls of residence. The three of us were covered in bruises. On arrival back in my office, I typed an account of the incident and released this over our Intranet. I affirmed that the students' actions would not deter us from our determination to restore decency and discipline to the University and from ensuring that the regulations of the University were upheld.

Apart from those whom I mentioned earlier, a number of other individuals tried to help me during the assault. Nick Igbokwe confronted Adenekan and ended up being threatened himself. He phoned the ASUU Chairman, Dr. H.C. Illoh, who said he was on his way to Akure and could not help. I heard that after the attack some ASUU leaders celebrated the event in the Staff Club with copious amounts of beer. A student, Victor Ado, confronted "Old Soldier," the student who had been kicking me continuously, and struggled with him to save me, and then got attacked himself. He was saved by Solomon Dada and Rotimi Odofin, who joined Victor in trying to rescue me. While I was lying on the ground, Rotimi Odofin took off my tie to prevent the attackers from strangulating me. Lateef Salami, a dental student, also tried to rescue me, but was overpowered by the mob. Victor Ado gave evidence against a number of the perpetrators, including "Old Soldier." He risked his life in doing so, and on 12 March 2005, he was attacked by "armed robbers" in the town. He frantically phoned me at about 3am that morning, and I contacted the Police. He escaped, more by luck or divine intervention. Two others who had come to my assistance during the assault, Solomon Dada and Rotimi Odofin, were also attacked by armed men in the town.

Immediately after we had been rescued, there was a confrontation between the students and the Police. The mob ran and retreated while my two companions and I, went back up to my office. The Police rescue team arrived just in the nick of time. At that point, I was not aware that the bus had been parked overnight on the campus. If we had been driven away, it would certainly not have been to Awolowo Hall. I am convinced that those who planned the incident had more deadly intentions for us.

Then came the real tragedy. The mob had retreated as far as the road outside Fajuyi Hall. There they confronted the Mobile Policemen. More tear gas was fired, and there were gun shots. A Part I student, Rasheed Laketu, was shot in the head. He was dead on arrival at the Health Centre. The subsequent autopsy revealed that the bullet came from a handgun. Soon after we arrived back in my office, we learnt that the student had been shot. I phoned the Director of Health Services, Dr. Aderounmu, who told me he was dead. I felt terrible. The sense of guilt over that young man's loss lives with me to this very day and will remain with me till I die. I visited his family the following weekend, accompanied by Professor Rahaman, a leader of the Muslim Community in the University. I told them what was in my heart:"When you sent your son to the University, you were entrusting his care and his safety to me, as Head of the University. I failed you." Their reaction overwhelmed me. In the midst of their grief, they showed understanding and compassion to me when I had expected only their anger and condemnation.

After the confrontation with the students, the Police retreated to the front of the Computer Centre. This allowed a small group of students to invade the University Hall. They could not get up to the offices, because the gates to the stairs had been locked. They entered the underground car park and vandalised a number of vehicles, including a number of the University's vehicles and my Pajero. Around that time, Wale Adebayo was ambushed by a small mob near the Library and brutally attacked. He was severely injured.

I issued an order closing the University and I reported this action to an emergency meeting of the University Senate the following evening. I prayed that, as had happened after the 10 July 1999 exodus, there would be no accidents on the road, and that all of the students would return safely to their homes.

The assault was reported to the Police, who declared some of the main perpetrators wanted. I set up an Investigation Panel chaired by Professor Eyo Okon of the Department of Zoology, a famous authority on bats. The Investigation Panel's work was protracted, because the University had been closed, and they did not have access to the majority of the witnesses and to those involved until the University re-opened in January 2005. The Panel's report identified 29 individuals as having a case to answer. In compliance with the University law, I ordered that 28 of them be brought before a Disciplinary Panel chaired by Professor Ogunkoya of the Department of Geography. In the case of Peter Olowokandi, there was no requirement for a Disciplinary Panel, since he had committed the offences in my presence. I expelled him for his gross misconduct and for failing to comply with his earlier suspension. It should be noted here that I did not cite any offence, such as assault, which would have been of a criminal nature and, which would have brought the offence outside the remit of the University, since criminal cases are required to be dealt with under the criminal justice system. Professor Ogunkoya's Panel reported in April. Based on the report, I ordered the expulsion of seven students, including Olawoyin, Adenekan, Aderibigbe ("Old Soldier"), and Adegbile. Two others were suspended for four semesters each. Incidentally, the three Students' Union officers who had come up to my office to rescue me were also recommended for disciplinary action for their part in initiating the demonstration, but I took no action against them in view of the circumstances. I actually expressed admiration for their courage in confronting Olowokandi and his mob. The Students' Union President, Mohammed Elegbede, played no part in the 3 November episode; once more, he had disappeared from the campus during the crisis. In July 2005, he was impeached by the Union for, among other things, his "failure to defend the interests of Great Ife students," but reinstated by its Judicial Commission on appeal.

We had taken very firm action against the perpetrators of the outrage on 3 November. However, the majority of those whom had been rusticated, including the ringleaders, did not vacate the campus and continued to fuel and engage in subversion. Adenekan, in particular, was to participate in another major student crisis, this time, a religious conflict.

Religious conflicts, particularly between Christians and Muslims, have been a feature of Nigerian life for many years. For most of its history, the University had not experienced any major problems, although there were undercurrents.

The first problem that I faced was not between Christians and Muslims, but within the Islamic religion. A minority of Muslims in the University are members of the Ahmadiya sect. This group is considered by the main Muslim Community to not be true Muslims. The students, under the umbrella of the Muslim Students' Society (MSS), were strongest in their antagonism of the Ahmadis, who had their own society. The MSS labelled the Ahmadis as "heretics." They had separate praying areas in the halls of residence, but used the main University Mosque on Fridays, to the resentment and sometimes the resistance of the main Muslim Community. Early in 2000, on two occasions, members of the MSS attacked the Ahmadi students in their headquarters office. In October, the same year, the Ahmadis organised a seminar, to be attended by members of the sect from all over the country. The MSS were infuriated at the plan, and vowed to resist it vigorously. A group of them attacked the Ahmadi students' office in Fajuyi Hall, assaulted those present, and removed all their property there. We interacted with both groups, but the MSS insisted that the seminar should not take place. The leaders of the Muslim Community also requested us to ban the seminar and repeated its advice that the Ahmadis should be denied recognition by the University. I refused, insisting that all religious groups should have the freedom to practice their beliefs. The seminar went ahead, heavily protected by the University's Security Service, without any major incident. We had informed the Police of the problem, but their assistance was not required. Thereafter, the Ahmadis were allowed to practice their religion, albeit to the resentment of the main Muslim Community.

One other problem that we had with the MSS was that a core of them appeared to hold, and practice, rather extreme views. This is not unusual among young people. From about 2000 onwards, a small number of female Muslim students started wearing the Niqab (or Burka), a black attire which included a full-mask face cover with a slit for the eyes and a long gown which hid everything except the hands and feet. The latter were often covered by socks. The numbers were initially small, but gradually increased. Academic staff began to raise an alarm, ostensibly because they could not identify those they were teaching in their lectures and, in particular, those they were examining in the examination halls. It is very likely that some of the protesting members of staff, Christians of extreme views, also had religious motives behind their objections. The Muslim Community was also against this full veiling. The Administration wanted to put a stop to this extremist form of dress, and we took the opportunity to draw up a dress code, approved by the Governing Council in February 2002, which covered other aspects of dress that were causing complaints, including the extremely provocative and seductive way in which some female students dressed. The Governing Council approved the dress code, but the MSS resisted it, and some of the female Muslim students continued to wear the burka. Some had to be sent out of class. Gradually, the practice petered out, although some still wore the burka outside the classroom.

A more worrying development was the discovery that some Muslim students were getting married to each other, getting pregnant, delivering their babies in the Awolowo Hall Mosque and living in the Mosque with their babies. We also had cases where female Muslim students, having adopted fundamentalism against the wishes of their parents, disowned their parents. In

August 2005, a parent reported to us that his daughter had been kidnapped. Unknown to her parents, the girl had gotten married to a fellow Muslim student, and refused to see her parents when they came to visit. When her father decided to take her home, she disappeared, aided and abetted by four MSS leaders, who spirited her away. The matter was reported to the Police, who declared the four students wanted. Eventually, with the assistance of the Muslim community, we were able to locate her and she reluctantly returned to her parents. However, she temporarily withdrew from the University because she insisted on wearing the Nikab to class.

The students of Great Ife have a culture of militancy. Historically, this is most often directed at the University Administration or the Government and its functionaries. At times, it has been directed against themselves. If there is no agency towards which they can direct their aggression, they sometimes turn it onto themselves. In the late morning of a Sunday in April 2004, I was fishing at the "Agric" dam, when up came the senior security officer on duty. He told me that they were faced with a serious problem in Mozambique Hall, a female hostel, and they could not handle it. I proceeded to the Hall, dressed in my shabby fishing clothes, to find a scene of absolute chaos. Earlier that morning, the students in the Hall had discovered a "peeping Tom". He had jumped over the fence and hidden himself nearby to observe the ladies bathing. He had been "arrested" and imprisoned in a room. The peeping Tom was an Awolowo Hall student, and when the news reached that hall, the Awo boys had mobilised to free him. The Awo boys had gone en masse to Mozambique Hall, joined on the way by a large contingent of male students from nearby Angola Hall. The ladies had locked themselves in, shouting taunts at the attackers. The shouting had degenerated into physical combat, with various missiles being flung from both sides. I had to go into the middle of the melée, with missiles flying around me. If I hadn't, the riot would have degenerated further. I was joined by *Bablo*. It took over an hour to restore sanity. I got the young voyeur released into the custody of the Security Department and the injured, mainly girls, were taken to the Health Centre. I set up a panel to look into the incident, but the main instigators of the conflict couldn't be identified. I disciplined the peeping Tom.

I believe that, as a result of the 3 November 2004 episode and the previous students' crises that had disrupted the University's academic programme, a groundswell of anti-militant opinion developed. Most students wanted peace in the University, and no further delays before they could graduate. A less confrontational Students' Union Executive was generally desired. A loose association of the Student Christian groups on the campus, called the University Joint Campus Mission (UJCM), put forward Olanrewaju Idowu, nicknamed "Diamond," who was seen as one of them. He had a landslide victory in the elections in June 2005. Several of the other members of the Executive were also pacifists, and did not belong to any of the militant political groups. Things were more peaceful for a while, but the former Students' Union leaders, and the political associations, in particular the Pacesetters, were still at work. A more serious problem was that "Diamond" allowed the militants in the student body to manipulate him.

As an illustration, one night we received information that the President had led some students to the Postgraduate Hall to forcibly take over some rooms on behalf of undergraduate students. I went to the scene with Wale Adebayo. We found a small mob of students creating chaos. The President was there, and so also were Adenekan and some of the Pacesetters group. Adenekan appeared to be effectively in charge, but quickly faded into the background. It then became clear that "Diamond" had lost control of the situation and did not know what to do next. Wale Adebayo started interacting with him, while I looked on. When the gravity of the situation was explained to him, "Diamond" lay down on the ground, signifying his helplessness. We drove all the invaders away through threats of disciplinary action and they all left. "Diamond" played no part in resolving the situation. This weakness in him was a major factor in the religious crisis that occurred towards the end of my term.

The final student crisis that I faced was fuelled by a religious conflict. I use the term "fuelled," because, as will be seen, the crisis was manipulated by some evil individuals. Shortly after midnight on 11 March 2006, a group of Muslim students went to the Awolowo Hall Common Room and confronted some students who were watching a pornographic movie there. They seized the video machine and the video cassette and took it to the Mosque, located in the former cafeteria of the hall. A large group of students then invaded the Mosque and attacked the occupants, injuring some, and causing some damage there. Informed over the radio, the Dean of Student Affairs, *Bablo*, Mr. Oduola, and some security officers, went to the scene and were able to restore order. They persuaded the Muslim students to return the seized video equipment. The showing of the pornographic movie resumed in the common room.

In the early hours of that morning, there was a loud bang near the Mosque. This was followed by a rapidly spreading rumour that firearms and ammunition were being stored in the mosque. The noise was interpreted as a gunshot; it was most certainly a firework, let off by some miscreants. A congress of the students was held in the Hall that morning, at which the claim that arms and ammunition were in the Mosque was discussed, and the congress resolved to enter the Mosque and investigate the claim. Warned of the development over the radio, Mr. Oduola and some security officers went to the Hall and entered the Mosque. They emerged and announced that they had found neither arms nor ammunition. By then, a large number of students had gathered outside. Mr. Oduola invited three student leaders, including the Students' Union President, to come in and see for themselves. The President, "Diamond" agreed, but Adenekan confronted him and insisted that they should all go in. "Diamond" changed his mind. The mob of students then invaded the Mosque once more. A battle ensued. The invaders were initially driven out by the Muslim students. The battle then continued outside. Things got out of hand. I was working in my office that morning. At around 10am a senior security officer came up to inform me of the problem, stating that the situation was out of control. I left for Awolowo Hall. As I was leaving, I met Biodun Adediran, the Deputy VC (Academic), who agreed to accompany me.

We arrived in Awolowo Hall to find it in an uproar. There was a pitched battle in the vicinity of the cafeteria, which housed the Mosque. The two sides, Muslims and the other group, were attacking each other with sticks, iron bars, and any other item that could serve as a weapon. Missiles were also being thrown, including stones, rocks, and even iron bars and planks. Bleeding combatants were lying on the ground. Members of staff from the Muslim Community, security staff, and Hall staff had all retreated after their efforts to stop the fighting had failed and because of the danger to themselves. However, I had no choice but to go into the middle of the melée and try to put a stop to the mayhem. I was in serious danger, because the missiles were flying all around me. It took several minutes for a number of us to separate the warring factions, by driving them back with threats of dire punishment as well as using sheer physical force. We won a breathing space, but with the tension still very high and both sides shouting threats and abuse at each other, and with missiles still being thrown. With the achievement of what was clearly a temporary lull, I requested two senior members of the Muslim Community, Professor Durosinmi and Dr. Yusuff, to get all the Muslims back into the Mosque, and when this became possible, to get them out through a rear exit. Although the Muslim students were in the Mosque and out of sight, the situation continued to be extremely tense. A large number of students from the various halls gathered outside the Mosque, shouting that Muslims should be evicted from the Hall. Eleven students required treatment for their injuries; the damage to the Hall and to property in the Hall was extensive.

We requested for a contingent of Mobile Policemen, who we stationed at the main gate of the University. In the afternoon and evening I held a number of consultations with various groups in the University, including the students. Although all of those consulted wanted the University to remain open, I could not obtain any convincing assurances that the conflict would not continue. Indeed, it was clear to me that there was a major danger that the situation would escalate. I ordered the immediate vacation of the University by all the students. They were to return ten days later, when the Harmattan Semester examinations would begin immediately. By tradition, it is the University Senate that has the prerogative of opening and closing the University, but the situation demanded immediate action. When I reported the matter to the Senate, my actions were approved. The students returned after the short break, and the examinations were incident-free. An Investigation Panel was set up to enquire into the incident. It produced wide ranging recommendations concerning religious activities in halls of residence and the academic area. Many of these recommendations were impracticable. For example, we implemented a recommendation banning religious services in the halls and lecture theatres. This left the various Christian splinter groups with nowhere to hold their weekly services. On the first Sunday after the ban was imposed, the various groups were milling about on the campus roads. We reversed that decision.

There was relative peace in the University until I left two months later.

The reader may well wonder why I got into these dangerous confrontations so often. I could certainly have avoided the personal confrontations. Indeed, in most of the incidents described above, I was advised to stay clear. There are a number of reasons why I did not "run away". First, I believe firmly that a VC who runs away from his students (or indeed his staff) has no business being a VC. I also must admit that I am stubborn as well as confrontational. I have never run away from anything. Dorothy Salami's rhetorical question "You like a fight, don't you?" is also relevant here. There were also situations where I just had to confront the danger. If I had not gone to the scene during the conflict at the Awolowo Hall Mosque, a tragedy would have occurred; some students would certainly have been killed. The most serious incident was certainly that of 3 November 2004. I was advised not to go to the office that day. However, the students had planned to confront me in the VC's Lodge if I had stayed away.

XVIII

Misadventures with ASUU

Industrial actions by ASUU have been relatively common over the last two decades. During my term in office, there were four such actions. The first was in late 1999. It was a national action which was called off after five weeks. In April 2001, a more protracted national strike took place. That industrial action commenced when the University was in the middle of its semester examinations. However, the local branch allowed the examinations to continue. These earlier industrial actions were in pursuit of a number of demands to the Government, including an improvement in funding the university system, university autonomy, and improvement in the conditions of service of academic staff. This last demand was actually the most important. In almost every case of industrial action in the universities, once the demand for increased pay was met, the more altruistic objectives tended to be forgotten. In June 2001, the industrial action by ASUU escalated, with an "all-out" strike. At that time Babalola Borishade was now the Minister of Education. He called all the VCs to a meeting in Abuja and directed us to stop the salaries of striking academic staff and open a register of those who were willing to work. The verbal directive was followed by a circular which stated that those on strike should not only lose their salaries but also lose their continuity of service. I ordered the Deans to open registers in every faculty. Less than 10% of the lecturers signed it. I did not stop salaries and, fortunately, the Government came to an agreement with the Union over their demands. At the same time, the Government also signed agreements with the other university unions, granting pay awards.

In November 2001, the University received the new salary scales, and was instructed to implement them. The new scales were implemented, and there was peace in the University. However, after only one month, we received a circular from the Ministry of Education which modified the mode of implementation of the new salaries in respect of the academic staff. The award was adjusted to provide for only a 22% increase, in basic salaries, rather than what had actually been agreed. The Government had agreed on a 22% salary increase, but ASUU had successfully negotiated on the basis of a differential of two steps between the salary scales of the academic over non-academic staff. The 22% was to be applied to this enhanced salary. The new directive was clearly an attempt by the Government to renege on its agreement, presumably to save money. I wrote to express concern over the new circular, and I presume some other VCs did the same, because it was certainly going to lead to industrial action. All the VCs were summoned to a meeting with the Minister in Abuja that month. Babalola Borishade, the Minister of Education stated unequivocally that the award to ASUU was 22% over their previous salaries, and this was to be implemented. Our protests were ignored; we were to implement the amended award.

I consulted with my colleagues in the Administration and it was decided that we had no choice but to implement the unilaterally amended award. I informed the Union of the position. At the same time, the other unions protested over the implementation of their own awards; I have never been able to understand why, since their awards were not modified. ASUU embarked on a five-day warning strike, and the other unions on a more protracted action. The University came to a standstill.

It will be recalled that in November 2000, the Governing Council had directed that the "No work, no pay" convention (it is actually a law in Nigeria) should be implemented for all future strike actions. Council had directed that this should not be implemented in respect of the April 2001 strike action in view of the manner in which ASUU had cooperated over the semester examinations. However, for the strike of 2002, I went ahead and stopped salaries for the period of strike action. For ASUU, this was only five days, but the period involved was longer for the other unions. The action was received with great hostility by the entire academic community. It should be noted here that, after I had implemented "No work, no pay" against NASU in 2000, that action had been enthusiastically endorsed by the University Senate, which had itself pronounced that this position should be implemented for all future strikes. When a member asked whether this would apply to strikes by academic staff, this was also endorsed by acclamation. Not so when they were faced with the reality. There was general uproar. I had enforced the position in respect of a strike action by SSANU a few months earlier. ASUU gave notice of strike action unless I reversed the decision.

Council met around that time, and set up a committee chaired by Professor Ijomah to seek a solution. Professor Ijomah's committee recommended that only the basic salaries should not be paid; the allowances (which actually accounted for the greater part of the take-home pay) would be paid. The Union accepted this. I protested vigorously, insisting that the law should be fully enforced. I was the only one with this view, but I spoke so forcibly that my position was accepted. This position was extremely foolish. Within days I had to reverse it. I attended an ASUU congress, and explained that the law needed to be applied in full so that "people would feel it," and that the action would put a stop to irresponsible industrial actions. I tried to imply that the "irresponsible actions" applied to NASU and SSANU, and not to strikes by academic staff. More foolishness. I left the congress in an atmosphere of great hostility. Many of those present were actually screaming abuse. I was in trouble. At that time, the Students' Union was very volatile. I was advised and I believed this to be the case, that if ASUU went on a further strike, they would also mobilise the students to cause major disruption, and that some of their leaders were capable of arranging that deaths would occur during the disturbances. I took advice from a group of senior academics, which included Dr. (now Professor) Yemi Mojola, whose opinion I greatly respected. Their advice was to back down. I phoned the Pro-Chancellor in a panic and got his agreement. It was total capitulation. Council had advised that only basic salaries should be withheld; in the end, nothing was withheld. The problem was solved, at least for the moment, but I had created much hostility towards myself among members of the academic staff.

The Government did not reverse its decision over the "two steps." Needless to say, ASUU decided to embark on national industrial action over this injustice. The initial action, which began in the first quarter of 2002, was to refuse to process examination results. The University was the first to be affected by the decision. We had just concluded the Rain Semester examinations, and the consequences were disastrous. The Faculty of Pharmacy and the College of Health Sciences insisted on concluding their examinations and processing the results. All the other Faculties refused to do so. As a result, final-year students could not go for National Youth Service, and were stuck in their homes for the following year, until results were finally released. Repeated entreaties to the Union did not change its rigid position. In March 2003, following an appeal, the local branch of the Union actually agreed to process the graduating students' results, but their decision was countermanded by the National Executive.

The industrial action was subsequently converted to an all-out strike in December 2002. Every federal university was closed. The Minister summoned the VCs to Abuja once more in January 2003. He directed that the "No work, no pay" law should be imposed on the striking members of staff, and handed over a written directive to that effect. I met with the ASUU Executive and informed them of the position. They stated that there would be serious consequences if they were not paid. They added that they were employed to provide teaching, research, and service, and they were still providing the latter two services. For this reason, they should be paid their salaries. This is an argument that they have advanced, time after time. It makes sense only to those who want to do no work and yet get paid! I have heard a further advance on this argument to the effect that after they do go on strike, when they return to work, all the subjects get taught eventually! The argument pays no heed to the effects of their actions on the lives of the young students whose futures are held to ransom. The University Senate, comprised wholly of ASUU members, repeatedly supported their Union's position.

The Government's position was wrong and grossly unfair. It had agreed to a new salary scale for the academic staff, circulated a pay structure along with this, and then reduced the award unilaterally. Thus, there was no doubt that the strike action by ASUU was justified. The Committee of VCs agreed with this position, although perhaps they did not articulate their support forcibly enough to the Government. At a meeting with the Minister of Education, Babalola Borishade, I stated this position, but he was unmoved; his argument was that the amended award was all that the Government could afford. The University's Governing Council agreed that an injustice had been perpetrated, and, to its credit, communicated this position to the Ministry in categorical terms. Professor Olikoye Ransome-Kuti had been appointed Chairman of the National Primary Health Care Development Agency, and I went to see him in Abuja. He was highly respected by the Government, and I felt he could intervene successfully. I explained the position and the extremely unfair action that followed, and requested him to intervene with the Government. He promised to discuss the matter with the President, although I did not receive any feedback from him subsequently. Shortly before that meeting, I had visited Professor Ransome-Kuti and informed him of the decision of the University to award him an honorary degree. He was delighted. Tragically, the Convocation ceremony at which the degree was to be conferred was postponed because of the strike. He died before the ceremony, and the degree had to be conferred posthumously.

At the end of November 2002, I visited Chief Gani Fawehinmi, one of the most famous Human Rights Lawyer in the country at that time and one of the most respected and influential individuals in ASUU circles, seeking his intervention. Gani received me very warmly. He listened very carefully to my position which was that a major injustice had been perpetrated on the academic staff but the victims of the industrial action were the students. He said he would consult with the ASUU President, Dipo Fasina. I felt very honoured by the courteous welcome Gani extended to me. He even showed me round his Chambers after our discussion. However, a week later, I received a ten-page letter from him containing his analysis of the position and concluding that ASUU was right.

The Federal Government backed up its directive that the striking members of staff should not be paid by stopping the subvention for salaries. SSANU and NASU also went on strike around this time; I cannot recall what this strike was about. The "No work, no pay" law was also applied to them. The Association of University Technologists of Nigeria (ASUTON) was not on strike, but funds were also not provided to pay their salaries. Things were extremely grim. We maintained water and power supply through the use of volunteers, but none of the other services was provided. The Government had stopped the subvention to all the universities in January 2003, but we had scraped together funds to pay that month's salaries because of an impending Muslim festival. Salaries were not paid between February and April 2003. One very controversial action that we took, and one which caused even more hostility, was that we were able to procure funds to pay individuals who could be considered to be working. I obtained the funds as a "Loan" after a meeting with Professor Peter Okebukola, the Executive Secretary of the National Universities Commission. I had explained that there were some members of the University who were working. The condition for release of the N100 million loan was that the money should not be used to pay individuals who were not working; I had to sign an undertaking to that effect. Those we paid included Deans and Heads of Department, who were certainly at work, and with whom the Administration was meeting regularly, and, of course, the technologists who were not on strike. The College of Health Sciences was also functioning more or less normally, and the students' clinical postings were continuing; they were also paid. I made an exception for the Head of Department of Physiological Sciences, Dr. Otas Ukponmwan, who was the Chairman of the ASUU branch in Ife, and who certainly was not working. Much more controversial was that we paid those who were providing the water and power supply. ASUU argued that this was not the normal function of those involved, and that the payments were "discriminatory." The hostility towards me got worse and worse. Most members of the University Community believed these "discriminatory" payments were wrong. However, none of those paid requested the University to withdraw the money from their accounts. In retrospect, I believe they were right, at least in respect of those academic and administrative staff assisting with power and water supply. Certainly, this action in paying some members of staff and not others greatly worsened the situation. ASUU, in particular, became even more determined to undermine my position. To them, I had become a pariah.

Everyone was suffering. Indeed, when salaries are delayed or not paid in the University the whole town suffers; the economy of Ile-Ife is heavily dependent on the University. ASUU and the other unions did not call off the strike until June. However, before then it had become clear that the University Community was fed up. In May, the Faculty of Pharmacy took a decision to go ahead with the final-year examinations, which had been suspended. The examinations were held, although a few of the lecturers refused to participate. SSANU and NASU called off their strikes. A meeting of the University Senate was called on 2 May to consider a recommendation from the Committee of Deans to re-open the University. ASUU met and resolved that the meeting should not take place. The Union picketed the Conference Centre, where Senate usually meets. One would normally expect that the picketing members of the Union would largely be relatively junior academics. This time, some professors joined in the picketing. Nevertheless, the members of Senate braved the situation and entered the meeting hall in spite of the anger and taunts of the picketing members of the Union. Shortly after the meeting commenced, two of the picketers, Professors Toye Olorode and O. Ajobo, entered the chamber carrying placards. They declared that the meeting was illegal, since ASUU, their Union, was on strike, and that we should all disperse. The Senate members ignored them. Professor Olorode then addressed me, repeating his claim about the illegality of the meeting, while Ajobo muttered abuse. I informed them that the meeting was going ahead and if they were not ready to participate in it, they could leave. They left. The meeting decided that the University should re-open, and that the outstanding examination results should be processed immediately.

Other universities were resuming academic activities. The Government resolved that the salaries of any university that was not fully functioning should continue to be withheld , and directed that the National Universities Commission should send teams to ascertain the situation in each institution. It would release funds for the payment of salaries to those universities that were functioning. We had a problem in that, apart from the College of Health Sciences and the Faculty of Pharmacy, the majority of the academic staff were not working. The team that came was headed by Professor M.A. Daniyan, the former VC of the Federal University of Technology, Minna, who was now working with the Commission. We had prepared well. We showed the team the academic activities in the College of Health Sciences and the Teaching Hospital, as well as the Faculty of Pharmacy, where the final year examinations were taking place. There were no academic activities in the other Faculties, but the team was very impressed by the activities surrounding the registration processes for returning students in these Faculties, which involved only the administrative staff and the Deans.

Thus we were able to convince the team that the University was fully at work, even though most of the members of the academic staff were in fact on strike. It was dishonest on our part, but we desperately needed to put an end to the suffering of the members of staff. Thus, the salaries for May were released and paid, even though the strike by ASUU was continuing in the University. Of course, we got no credit for this. The members of staff continued to smart from the three months' salaries that had not been paid, and, in particular, from the "discriminatory" payments to some individuals.

The strike was officially called off in June 2003, but the University's problems, and my problems, had only just begun. Worse was to follow. The University resumed, but the resentment over the events of the strike festered. All the unions insisted that their members should be paid for the three months from February to April. They bolstered this with the argument that the "discriminatory" payments to some members of staff were wrong, and that justice demanded that everyone else should be paid. In September 2003, at the end of the Harmattan semester, the local branch of ASUU formally declared that its members would not mark the semester examinations or process the results until the withheld salaries were paid. The examinations were concluded and the students left for the semester break, but no examination results were released except for those of the College of Health Sciences. Once more, our graduating students could not go for the Youth Service. The University could not reopen at the end of the vacation, because the results that were needed to register for the subsequent session were not available. As recorded in the preceding chapter, the situation with the students was extremely volatile. Re-opening under such circumstances would have resulted in turmoil from the student body.

The other universities were functioning normally but we were closed. At meetings of the Committee of VCs, all the members stated that they had not paid the outstanding salaries, and that the staff in their institutions were continually demanding for them. They expressed their sympathy for my situation. I later found that, one by one, they had all paid their staff and kept quiet about it in order not to arouse the wrath of the Government; the President, Olusegun Obasanjo, was known to have personally insisted that the salaries should not be paid.

The stalemate went on for almost a year. The Governing Council intervened repeatedly, appealing to the Union to soften its stance. The funds had been withheld by the Government and money was not available to pay the withheld salaries. However, funds were not the only problem; another major problem emanated from my position that the University must take a stand against such blackmailing tactics. ASUU was using the future of young people as its weapon. Our students were stagnating in limbo. The graduating class was once again unable to go for Youth Service; one whole year of their lives was lost. I believed that to capitulate to such weapons was to send a message that such evil acts could be rewarded. I held this position rigidly, at least at first. I recall that the Dean of Arts, Professor Sola Akinrinade, came to see me one night in the VC's Lodge, expressing his concern over the effects of the crisis on the future of the University he loved. I expressed my despair over the situation and then said, "If we yield to ASUU's demands we would have shown that evil can triumph." To this day, I maintain that the action of our ASUU branch in withholding the examination results was evil. I received a number of letters from alumni of the University and the parents of our students, all expressing deep concern over our continued closure. I replied to each one, giving a full explanation of the situation and the position of the University. I also met with the National Executive of the Alumni Association, who, concerned as they were, showed a remarkable level of understanding. The University Senate took up ASUU's position. At every meeting, it would affirm that the withholding of the salaries was wrong and they should be paid.

In September 2003, the Governing Council re-affirmed its support of the Federal Government's position on "No work, no pay." However, "in the interest of peace," it approved a "Special Council Grant" equivalent to one month's salaries to all the staff (except, of course, those who had already received the "discriminatory" payments). ASUU did not yield. It insisted that the entire amount should be paid. ASUU then entered a suit against the University and me in the Federal High Court in Osogbo in July 2004. The suit requested the Court to order the University to pay the two months' salaries that had been "illegally" withheld by the University. I took the advice of our very capable Legal Officer, Mrs. Ronke Ajibola, and we entered a counter-suit on behalf of the University requesting that the Court should order the lecturers to release the withheld examination results. Readers who are familiar with legal processes will know that these two suits were going nowhere. Following the institution of the University's suit, the Court joined both suits. After a number of hearings, the Judge advised both parties to settle out of Court. The University was advised to pay the outstanding salaries and the lecturers to process and release the results of graduating students. Both parties were to report on the proposed settlement at the next hearing. In fairness to ASUU, they did process the graduating students' results immediately afterwards. The University could not accede to the advice of the Judge; we did not have the money. Also, I must admit that at that time I was still dead set against paying the withheld salaries. On the University's part, I did write to the Minister of Education requesting permission to pay the withheld salaries and for the Ministry to release the required funds. I did not receive a reply. When the Court sat on the matter again on 8 October 2004, the lawyers for ASUU presented a notice to hold me in contempt of Court; the Judge gave me three months for a response, and subsequently advised our Legal Officer in his Chambers that I was in danger of being imprisoned on a charge of contempt of court. In the end, nothing came of this; the case petered out.

The impasse continued, I gradually began to change my rigid position. More and more people whom I trusted were advising that a compromise be reached. I was particularly worried about the effects of the continued closure of the University on its future and reputation. I actually feared that the crisis could even result in the death of the University. My tenure as VC was being marked more and more by crises and closures. It became increasingly clear that the University Administration could not win. We would have to pay the outstanding two months' salaries. However, even if we wanted to pay, the funds were not there. We had managed to pay the Council Special Grant, and had soon afterwards received a letter from the NUC to the effect that the money would be deducted from subsequent subventions; I wonder how the NUC found out about it.

The term of the Governing Council came to an end in July 2004. For nine months, we had no Governing Council and affairs that should concern the Council were handled by the Ministry of Education. We knew that there was no way that the Ministry would approve the payment of the outstanding salaries. However, we had decided that as soon as a new Council was appointed, we would request it to approve the payment of the money. We met repeatedly with the ASUU executive and gave an undertaking to recommend that Council should approve the payment of the two months' salaries as soon as it was reconstituted. I gave this undertaking in writing. No dice. The University remained closed.

A new Governing Council, under Professor S.J.S. Cookey, was appointed in April 2005. Professor Cookey had served two four-year terms as VC of the University of Port Harcourt, and was extremely knowledgeable about the University system. I went to see him in Port Harcourt as soon as his appointment was announced. I briefed him on the situation, and requested that, as soon as Council met, it should approve the payment of the withheld salaries. I also informed him of the Senate's decision that the University should be reopened. He advised that the University should not be reopened until the crisis was resolved, and agreed that, once the Council was formally inaugurated, it should deal with the outstanding salaries as a priority. He was true to his word.

During its first meeting in May 2005, the new Council agreed that the money should be paid and directed that the Administration should seek the funds to effect the payment according to a phased programme, with a minimum of N60 million a month. All the unions rejected the offer. The

Pro-Chancellor travelled down to the University and held a series of meetings with the unions and the Administration, at the end of which it was agreed that a more expeditious payment of the withheld salaries be effected; the Administration was to find the funds at all cost. The results were released immediately thereafter, and the University re-opened. We gradually scraped funds together, mainly by borrowing from accounts that were committed to other purposes, and eventually paid the outstanding salaries between June and August 2005. There was peace at last.

The crisis had been resolved, but only after the University, apart from the College of Health Sciences, had remained closed for one year. The reputation of the University suffered considerably. Most importantly, a whole year had been lost from the lives of our students. Our graduating students had not been able to participate in the National Youth Service for a whole year. The image of the University had suffered greatly. Many parents became reluctant to allow their children to apply for admission to Ife. We lost a lot of our friends in the process of this crisis. Can you imagine the response when you go to a company director, seeking support for a university project, when his children are at home instead of in school? The conflict was ostensibly between the Academic Staff Union and the University Administration: actually, it was between ASUU and I. However, the major victims were our students, and, of course, the University. The Administration, or should I say, I, Roger Makanjuola, made major mistakes in dealing with this crisis. While other universities were discreetly paying the salaries of their staff, we were holding rigidly to the Government's position. However, I must state here, once more, that my real objection was to the strategy of ASUU in using the lives and future of our students as their weapon of warfare. The first mistake was in confronting ASUU in a conflict that we could not win. They were too strong and too determined. The second mistake was in sticking to our guns in the face of an increasingly untenable position, thus prolonging the crisis and the suffering. After the withheld salaries were paid, Professor Okebukola, the Executive

Secretary of the NUC, confronted me in his office. I admitted that the salaries had been paid. He expressed surprise and disappointment. I replied that I had been presiding over the death of the University that I loved, and could see no other way out. He appeared to understand. I was subsequently informed that, when he learnt of our action, President Obasanjo was furious.

Earlier on in this book, I have expressed the belief that we were able to deal with NASU and SSANU effectively. Their teeth were drawn because we had deprived them of their major weapons of violence, sabotage of installations and deprival of services to the community. The same cannot be said of ASUU.

Professor Cookey arrived on the scene less than a year before my term as VC ended. He must take a lot of the credit for resolving the crisis. I greatly admired him. As I stated earlier, he had an admirable grasp of the university system and was committed to making the University work. He brought in innovations that enhanced the standards of the institution. I believed that he was also very supportive of me, although I was extremely disappointed when I found that he had been meeting with ASUU as well as student leaders behind my back. I have it on good authority that when discussing the crisis over the withheld salaries with the ASUU executive, he had stated: "The VC is the problem."

XIX

Making Progress

¤ ¤ ¤ ¤ ¤ ¤ ¤ ¤ ¤ ¤ ¤

In 1999, the University had only one emeritus professor, Professor Isaac Adeagbo Akinjogbin. Professor Adesanya Grillo, who had occupied our other emeritus chair, died in 1998. We processed three new emeritus chairs through Senate and Council in November 2003. These were Professor Wole Soyinka, Professor David Ijalaye of International Law, and Professor Gabriel Makanjuola of Agricultural Engineering. I was particularly pleased about Professor Soyinka. It took me three years to persuade him to accept the appointment and then to process the application. The emeritus appointment of Nigeria's only Nobel Laureate brought great kudos to the University, and we certainly capitalised on it. Professor Soyinka spent very little time in the University, but having him on our books was good enough. He provided support to our efforts in the area of cultural studies and agreed to direct the second revived International Festival of the Arts, though this did not eventually take place until after I had left.

One of the major objectives of the founding fathers of the University was the promotion and study of African cultures. This particular area had been on the back burner for a while.

We gave priority to its revival. The first capital project that we embarked on was the completion of the abandoned Institute of Cultural Studies building. Another related project, a museum of antiquities being developed by Chief John Odeyemi, had also been abandoned. I met with Chief Odeyemi, and he agreed to resuscitate the project. True to his word, work recommenced. I advised him to amend the designation of the museum and the Martin Aworinlewo Odeyemi Museum of Antiquities and Contemporary African Art was finally commissioned in April 2004. It was named after Chief Odeyemi's late father. It was stocked with a number of valuable exhibits, both antiquities and contemporary items, some of which are truly beautiful. These included a set of Gelede regalia, which formed the main initial exhibit. Unfortunately, up till the time of writing, environmental control of the exhibits has not been provided for the museum. I fear for the health of our valuable exhibits.

Professor Ola Rotimi, who had left Ife in the 1970s for the University of Port Harcourt before moving to the United States, returned to the University in 1998. One of his first achievements was to attract a Ford Foundation grant for an Ife Outreach Project. A team was set up to organise the project. I was the chairman. We were all truly excited over the project. This was a major, two-week long programme of performances, workshops, and seminars which were to take place in the University and in the town. On the morning of 18 August 2000, the Planning Committee were gathered in a committee room on the ground floor of the University Hall, waiting for Ola Rotimi's arrival when someone came into the room to announce that the playwright had been found dead an hour before.

I drove to his isolated home on the Ife-Ede road with Professor Olomola, the Director of the Institute of Cultural Studies. We entered the house to find Ola Rotimi, lifeless, lying on the floor of his bedroom. He appeared to have suffered a fatal stroke during the night. So passed away one of Nigeria's greatest playwrights. The tragedy was particularly great for the University because we had looked to him to revitalise Cultural Studies in Ife. After his funeral, we met with officials of the Ford Foundation, who agreed that the Ife Outreach Project should go ahead. Professor Olomola and his team organised it very successfully in August 2001. There were a number of activities which involved academics and other interested parties from all over Nigeria during the project. However, I believe the true impact of the project came from the performances and workshops. Troupes came from all over the country, and some of the performances were truly spectacular. These performances were organised in various parts of the town, as well as in the University. Most were outdoors on a mobile stage that was specially constructed for the programme. Renowned experts held workshops to provide hands-on training in various traditional arts and crafts. These experts included the sculptor, Lamidi Fakeye, the musicologist, Tunji Vidal, and the only remaining bronze caster in Ife, Chief Oluyemi. Oluyemi actually constructed a bronze foundry, which has remained a permanent fixture of the Institute of Cultural Studies. The impact of this project on the University was significant—Ife was, once more, on the cultural studies map of the world.

Much credit goes to Professor Olomola who did a fine job in resuscitating Cultural Studies in the University. An increasing number of cultural programmes were organised, the academic programmes were invigorated, and Ife, the journal of the Institute, resumed regular publication. Professor Olomola retired in 2004 so a new Director was required. Wale Adeniran represented the Faculty of Arts on the Board of the Institute, on which I was chairman. I had been extremely impressed by his ideas for developing the Institute. He was at that time a Lecturer Grade I, but I felt he could do the job. Biodun Adediran, who was the Deputy VC (Academic) at the time, and whose advice I valued, agreed with me. Much to the annoyance of the various professors in the institution who felt that they were better qualified for the job, I appointed Wale as Acting Director. Wale's appointment heralded a further upliftment of the Institute and of cultural activities in the University. He is a truly gifted and committed academic, and he also brought innovation and brilliance to the leadership of the Institute. I was truly delighted with his efforts.

In April 2005, Wale came to my office with some visitors from the Republic of Benin. The visitors were the leadership of the Association Internationale Groupe Gelede. Gelede had recently been designated as an intangible cultural heritage by UNESCO, largely as a result of the efforts of this group. They were interested in promoting an exhibition on Gelede in the University. We were delighted. In its earlier history, the University had organised an Annual Festival of Arts and Culture, which had achieved international status. The Festival had last taken place in 1985. Wale and I had been discussing the resuscitation of the Festival. This was a grand opportunity, and we agreed to revive the event around a Gelede Festival. The team from the Republic of Benin agreed. Wale went about raising funds, mainly from local benefactors, prominent among whom were Chief John Odeyemi and the Ooni of Ife. The Festival took place from12 to18 May 2005 and was a spectacular success. Apart from the exhibition and performances of Gelede, there were academic activities and other cultural performances. The Ife International Festival of Arts and Culture had returned after 20 years. We planned to make the Festival an annual event, and Wole Soyinka agreed to direct the next one. Unfortunately, it had to be postponed because of the political events in the country. The second edition of the Festival did not take place until 2008.

As a result of the instability and turmoil in the University, honorary degrees had not been awarded since the early 1990s. In 2002, we processed the awards of six honorary degrees. I was particularly delighted that among those honoured were my mentor, Olikoye Ransome-Kuti, Mr. David Adeyanju, a local businessman who had done so much for the Ile-Ife community, and our Chancellor, the Emir of Katsina, who I regarded as a truly great and likeable individual. I was also very excited that an honorary Doctor of Laws degree was to be conferred on Gani Fawehinmi. Gani, who died in 2009, is, in my opinion, one of the greatest Nigerians who ever lived. He gave me much personal support. He was very popular in the University because of his courageous sacrifices in the cause of human rights and his support of both ASUU and the students during their struggles.

He was a major thorn in the flesh of successive Governments and I do not believe any other university would readily have given him an honorary degree. It says a lot for the University that we unhesitatingly decided to give him the award, in spite of our knowledge that the Government would not like it. The awards were not conferred until 2003 because of the ASUU industrial crisis. By then, Olikoye and David Adeyanju had died. Their awards were conferred posthumously, received on their behalf by Bose, Beko Ransome-Kuti's wife, and Gbenga, David Adeyanju's son. In 2005, we conferred honorary degrees on four individuals. These were Justice Fati Lami Abubakar, a truly remarkable lady and alumnus of the University; Professor Mario Radicella of the Institute of Theoretical Physics in Trieste, Italy, who had been instrumental in the development of ICT in the University; the renowned Public Health academic, Professor Adetokunbo Lucas, and Raymond Zard, an Ibadan businessman and philanthropist. Ife lived up to its reputation of conferring honorary degrees only on individuals who truly deserved it, and not because of any benefits or ulterior motives for the institution. I can say with pride that we are the only university in the country that has that enviable reputation.

The greatest challenge that the University faced during my tenure was funding. This problem was common to all the Federal universities in the country.

The first Nigerian university, the University of Ibadan, was established by our former Colonial Government in 1948. Although the students paid modest fees, the institution was funded almost entirely by the Government. The managers were able to provide excellent facilities without any anxiety over the finances provided by the Government. Even after independence, this situation of financial buoyancy continued. Three new universities were established in the early 1960s, and these institutions were also able to function, and function well, almost entirely on Government funding. The University of Ife, now the Obafemi Awolowo University, was one of these, and its proprietors, the Government of the Western Region, provided admirably for the needs of the institution. It should also be noted that, in those early days, there was substantial support from external agencies, mainly from America and Britain.

Many more universities were established in the 1970s, mainly by state governments, but in 1975 they were all taken over by the Federal Government, which at that time was so enriched from the oil boom that the then Head of State could pronounce with confidence that "Money is not our problem but how to spend it"! Indeed, the Federal Government cancelled all tuition fees and pegged accommodation charges at N90.00 (at that time equivalent to US$110) per session. The oil boom was soon followed by severe economic decline, and the level of funding to the universities progressively decreased. The financial difficulties were compounded by the fact that provision now had to be made for so many universities from the nation's diminished resources.

The economic crunch, accompanied by political instability, set up a spiral of decline, the most important of which included:

- Social and moral decline within the university communities, which was a reflection of the situation in the larger society.
- The non-availability of development, maintenance and running costs; in particular, academic and research facilities became inadequate and of a poor standard.
- The collapse of the Naira, with a consequent deterioration in the standard of living of staff and students.
- The departure of expatriate staff and students, resulting from the above, and leading to the loss of the universities' international flavour—this was particularly so in Ife, which had attracted large numbers of staff and students from all over the world.
- Industrial and student unrest.

The financial crisis in the university system, in turn, contributed to additional problems. The morale of the university community was greatly affected so that our commitment to academic advancement and excellence also declined. The ideals that we used to share—dedication to teaching, advancing the frontiers of knowledge and making a true impact on the development of our local community and the nation—were no longer important. Who can blame the young lecturer who has to house, feed and educate his children if he looks to these challenges first?

What is the way forward? I believe that the first challenge is to address the financial crisis. If we alleviate the financial crisis, the other problems would also be partly alleviated. In addressing the financial crisis, we need to accept the following:

- The Government cannot provide the entire funding requirements of the university system.
- The universities need to raise funds to complement Government's subventions. This is the situation all over the world. The leading universities in the United States do not receive any direct government funding at all, except through research grants and services contracted by the government. The so-called state universities in the USA receive, on average, only 30% of their financial requirements from their state governments. Universities in Britain do receive a higher proportion, but still have to generate 35–50% of their requirements.

The alternative sources of funding include:

- Fees for tuition and other services to students
- Commercial activities
- Sponsored research
- Endowments
- Fundraising for development

Fees: There are few countries in the world where university education is free. In most countries that boast of so-called "free education", that education is funded through heavy taxation. In Nigeria we pay minimal taxes. If we want "free" education and "free" health care, we must be ready to pay appropriate rates of taxation. If we are not prepared to pay taxes, then we must be prepared to pay directly to subsidise the education and health of our children. There is one caveat here, which is that no person should be deprived of the opportunity of education just because they cannot pay for it. Bursaries, scholarships and loans need to be provided, not just for the gifted individual but also for the genuinely poor.

Commercial activities: The scope of commercial activities is diverse. They include investments and the provision of services. However, the greatest potential comes through the exploitation of our academic skills. All academic disciplines have enormous commercial potential, through consultancies, direct services, e.g., medical, fine art contracts, biographies, etc. and, in particular, the marketing of intellectual property. Emeritus Professor G.A. Makanjuola's mechanical yam pounder is probably the best example of this for Great Ife. There should have been many more by now. The academic and technological skills within the University have the potential to yield millions of dollars if properly exploited. Our problem is that we lack not just the awareness of our potential, we also lack the required marketing skills. This is where those in the private sector should come in. We need to join hands with them. We have the technical know-how and they have the business know-how.

University Advancement: The term "University Advancement" covers a number of fundraising activities. Most commonly, it covers development fundraising, sponsored research, endowments, legacies and annual gifts. The greatest resource (and greatest potential source of funds) of any university is its alumni, thus making alumni relations the an integral part of any advancement structure. Communications (or public relations) is an obviously important component of advancement activities. In my opinion, intellectual property and commercial enterprises should also be classified as advancement activities.

More and more Nigerian universities are now establishing advancement or development offices. This University's Advancement Office was established in April 2006, just before I left.

Resolving the financial crisis in the University is essential to the future of the institution. There are some other essential steps if we are to develop (or restore) the University to its position as a reputable, internationally recognised institution. We have to restore academic standards and discipline in the university system. Determined leadership is essential for this, drawing upon the core of committed academic and other staff who maintain their integrity and uphold the values of hard work, honesty, and honour.

It must be stated, once more, that the universities must give priority to generating their own income—that is the path to true autonomy and the path to survival. Our introduction of relatively modest charges to the students, which we succeeded in implementing in the face of major crises, has been described earlier.

Right from the beginning, we were aware of the great potential of philanthropic fundraising. We determined to give priority to advancement activities. However, we were faced with a number of problems. The protracted series of crises and the resulting closures greatly damaged the image of the University. There was also a perception within the country that Ife was not an exception to the apparent decline in the standards within the university system. Donors are attracted by success, and not by failure. The University had also failed to maintain contact with its friends, who, in many cases, had become disenchanted with the institution. The University community was generally not interested in the idea; indeed, many rejected it. Universities are conservative institutions, and the first generation of Nigerian universities, including Ife, is particularly conservative. The concept of fundraising was alien to most of us. Indeed, most members of the academic community held firmly to the belief that it was not their responsibility but that of the Government to fund the University. The "Ivory Tower" mentality was predominant; university staff believed that their places were in the laboratories and classrooms, and not out with what they perceived to be the begging bowl. This position was held even by most of the University's leadership, including the Deans. Finally, and possibly most important, I, the Chief Executive of the institution, had no clue how to go about fundraising, nor had any of my colleagues in Administration.

I mentioned earlier that the University had lost virtually all of its friends. A major exception was provided by the alumni. Right from the beginning of my tenure as VC, the Alumni

Association was extremely supportive, and clearly committed. I met with the National Executive soon after I resumed office, and also took every opportunity to meet with them and speak at meetings of its branches. My first effort at fundraising was directed at them. I requested their assistance in rehabilitating the halls of residence, which were in a terrible state, giving various options, such as making donations of building materials, making direct donations of funds, or taking on projects. Each time I made the request, the verbal response appeared positive, but nothing came in. Throughout my period of service, I worked to enhance the relationship of the Administration with the Alumni (actually, it was mainly their relationship with me). I attended as many meetings of the Association and its branches as I could, and each time I emphasised their importance to the University. I must say that I did have an excellent relationship with the alumni. However, initially, at least, their support was mainly moral rather than material.

A major breakthrough came with the election of Dele Oye as President of the Alumni Association in 2000. I had looked on him with suspicion when he was initially elected. He had mobilised a large number of previously inactive alumni to attend the National Convention to vote him in, and had spent a huge sum on their accommodation and transport. My sentiments had been in support of the candidate of a more socialism-oriented group from Lagos, among whom was Mr. Olumide-Fusika, whom I had come to admire during his representation of the students at the Judicial Commission. Dele Oye proved to be the best Alumni President the University has ever had, and it will be very difficult for any future alumni leader to surpass his achievements. He brought to the Presidency a remarkable degree of ability as well as commitment. Dele has a very successful law practice in Abuja. So committed was he that he spent his personal money on projects and also spent generous amounts to support alumni who were in difficulty. Under his Presidency, the two-storey Alumni Hall, a 56-bed female hostel, was constructed. This building was particularly remarkable in that it was the only two-storey building to be constructed in the

University since the 1980s; financial considerations had made bungalow structures the order of the day. Half of the cost of that building came from Dele Oye's pocket. We got on extremely well. We shared the same priorities as far as the University was concerned, and this included fundraising. Under his leadership, the Alumni organisation became an extremely strong body, with a membership that was deeply committed to the University and its development. The number of branches within the country almost doubled, and these were branches that were actively contributing to the image of the University as well as providing more practical support. It was during his time that the Alumni began to develop an international presence.

The international expansion of the Alumni organisation began through serendipity. During the NASU strike of 2000, I was working alone in my office when two individuals came up and introduced themselves as alumni from the United States of America. They were Eddy Olafeso and another alumnus. They were very much concerned about the crisis in the University and wanted to help. I explained what was happening and we had a long discussion about the industrial crisis and its causes. As the meeting went on, what struck me most about these two alumni was the great love that they had for "Great Ife." They wanted desperately to help and we started a discussion of their forming an overseas branch of the Alumni Association. They said there were many alumni living and working in Houston, USA, where they themselves lived, and that they themselves lives, and that they had actually registered an alumni association the year before but taken no further action. They said they would meet with these other alumni when they got back there and consider incorporating the association. Some weeks later I received an e-mail from Gbenga Agboola stating that "The Great Ife Alumni Association Association" had been incorporated, with Mrs. Yemi Koyejo, a petroleum engineer, as President. Their inaugural convention took place in August that year, and the Association provided my air ticket to attend the event in Houston. The event made a big splash; they also raised a substantial donation for the University. They have been holding these conventions every year since then, re-named the International Reunion. I attended the second one and Kwashi Ako-Nai attended the third, in 2003, where Chief Ernest Shonekan, a former Head of State, was the Guest of Honour. A Dallas branch was established in 2003. I had a meeting with the alumni in the Baltimore/Washington area when I attended a training programme in 2005; they agreed to establish a branch, but this was never formalised, and they continued to work with the larger group in Houston. These USA branches became an increasing source of support to the University. The enthusiasm of its members for their alma mater was truly impressive.

The alumni in the United Kingdom were not quite as active, but did organise low key activities and some financial support to the University. The medical alumni were the most prominent and I attended a luncheon in Newton Abbey when I was on leave in the UK in 2005.

Our first major fundraising project at home was the launching of a Development Fund, which we originally proposed to be organised around the University's Fortieth Anniversary in 2002. Although the University initiated this, the Alumni Association joined in wholeheartedly, and actually took the lead in some aspects. What follows is basically a description of how not to go about fundraising. As will be seen later, we did everything wrong and, indeed, everything went wrong. The first setback was that, because of the closure of the University as a result of the protracted industrial actions by the unions, the Convocation and the launch had to be postponed by one year. The event was eventually organised only three months after the University had re-opened, when the crisis was still fresh in everyone's mind. We drew up a list of prospective donors which included the Governors of the seven states that made up the former Western Region which had established the University, wealthy individuals with a history of a relationship with the University and some wealthy prospects just because they were wealthy. Teams from the University covered the entire nation, drumming up support. I headed the teams that visited the major prospects. We were invariably well received, with promises to participate in the event and vague promises of financial support, but with no real commitment in most cases. We were visiting prospective donors who had virtually no knowledge of us; in many cases they did not know any of us personally. People do not give under such circumstances; as you will see later, the cultivation and involvement of prospects are essential to philanthropic fundraising. Equally important was that the crisis in the University, whereby the children or grandchildren of these prospective donors had been stuck at home for over a year, was still fresh in their minds. The launch was to be the beginning and end of the appeal; we expected that all the funds would be raised on that day. No donations were sought in advance of the event, and we only received vague pledges. We identified an extremely wealthy alumnus as a prospective Chief Launcher and I headed a team to go out and meet him. We did not have an appointment, but travelled to Lagos nonethess in hope. We went to three of his companies before eventually locating his house, where we were fortunate to find him. None of us had ever met him. However, he received us well. He was in an expansive mood, and he agreed there and then to be Chief Launcher. We had a Chief Launcher, but we had no idea what his donation was going to be.

We put so much effort into the Development Fund Appeal. We were confident that there would be a proportional relationship between the level of these efforts and the funds raised. The branches of the Alumni Association held a number of events, mainly lunches and dinners, to raise funds. The yields were very modest, but we failed to regard this result as a premonition of the likely outcome of the main event.

The Ceremony on 6 December 2003 was truly memorable and spectacular. We began with the award of postgraduate diplomas and degrees, accompanied by speech after speech. We then went on to the award of the six honorary degrees, accompanied by more speeches. Gani Fawehinmi's degree was received with particular enthusiasm, especially by the students. We were all extremely happy. But by then, three hours had already passed. We then went on to the "Alumni Awards," whereby the Alumni Association gave awards to a substantial number of its members, accompanied by more speeches. Needless to say, by the time the Development Fund Appeal was launched, we had lost half of our audience, and those who remained were fed up. The Chief Launcher made his speech, followed by a donation of N5 million. A few others donated smaller amounts. This was meant to be a N500 million Development Fund!

Follow-ups with the various prospects yielded some additional funds. The largest donation came from the Government of Osun State. The Governor, Prince Olagunsoye Oyinlola, had proposed that the seven governments that made up the former Western Region should combine efforts to invest in a substantial project. When his efforts failed, he finally approved a donation of N10 million. In fact, Prince Oyinlola was the only one of the governors with whom we had developed a relationship prior to the event. A major cause of our failure was ignorance of the principles of philanthropic fundraising. The arrival of the Carnegie Corporation changed all that.

In 2002, I received an email from Andrea Johnson of the Carnegie Corporation of New York. The Corporation had formed a consortium of three America-based funding agencies to support the development of universities in Africa. The other agencies were the Macarthur Foundation and the Rockefeller Foundation. Andrea was the Programme Officer of the Carnegie Corporation on the initiative. The email provided some information on the programme and stated that the OAU was one of eight Nigerian institutions that had been identified as possibly having the required qualifications for support. We were invited to provide information and proposals on behalf of the University. I responded immediately, and over the next few weeks, provided a write-up on the University and a number of other documents. Later that year, a two-person team from the Corporation arrived, comprising Andrea and Professor Narciso Matos, the Director of the Africa Section of the Carnegie Corporation. The visit lasted four days. We showed them round the University. The team met with the University Administration and various groups, which included representatives of the female members of the academic staff, the Students' Union Executive, female students and the

ASUU Executive. The meeting with the ASUU executive was particularly eventful. The Executive was initially hostile, and the members expressed their suspicions of the motives of the funding agency, and indeed of all other such agencies from overseas. I was not surprised. The Union was at that time extremely hostile to international funding agencies. I had initially thought the hostility was towards the World Bank and the International Monetary Fund, which ASUU claimed were colluding with the Government to commercialise the educational system and control it. In 2002, Bill Saint, a Director of the World Bank, had been physically assaulted by staff and students in the University of Ibadan and ejected from the campus when he came to discuss the Bank's proposed support of the university. I had thought that there would be less hostility to philanthropic agencies. However, in the same year, a team from the Macarthur Foundation had been forcibly ejected from our campus by members of ASUU. My subsequent interactions with members of ASUU, very senior members at that, indicated that their suspicions extended also to the philanthropic agencies. They believed that the agencies had ulterior motives and that they were part of a sinister plot between the American and Nigerian governments to take over and control the educational system. The claim sounds ludicrous, but this was what they believed.

At the meeting, The ASUU delegation hardly allowed the team to explain the reasons behind their visit before they launched into an attack. Two interactions will illustrate this. One ASUU member said, "We know you will insist on including a programme on AIDS." Narciso replied "The decision is yours as to which projects you apply for. If you want us to fund a programme on AIDS we will consider it, but your university is to decide on what projects to apply for." The team did state that they would require a programme on Gender Equity to be included in the funding programme, and that all the other projects should take cognisance of gender equity. To this, Toye Olorode responded, "What is all this about gender when teachers are not being paid their salaries?" The confrontation continued for over an hour; the Carnegie team defended their position with calmness and reason. Gradually the hostility of the ASUU team thawed, and, in the end, they gave their support to the Carnegie Corporation's proposals, albeit half-heartedly. At the end of the four-day visit, the team was obviously impressed. We were invited to submit proposals for projects which would enhance the University's functions; they were termed development projects. The amount available was $2 million. A project to promote gender equity had to be included, and the other projects had to provide adequately for gender equity.

We invited proposals from the University community and vetted them. We ended up with nine projects that we believed would benefit the University and meet the Carnegie Corporation's criteria. We had to eliminate one of these because the $2 million would not cover all nine. Our team developed a concept paper in conjunction with individual project teams. This was approved by the Corporation, with extensive comments, and the teams were requested to develop the full proposals. The final proposal was submitted and approval came in May 2003. We had made it. Two million US dollars!

The approval was a great boost to our morale and to the image of the University. Of the eight Nigerian universities identified by the Carnegie Corporation as prospects for its support, only three, Ife, Jos and Zaria, had succeeded. The projects made a major impact on our services. The major part of the ICT development in the University during my term as VC was funded by that grant. In addition, a state-of-the art computer engineering laboratory was developed. The Central Science Laboratory was further developed and a second analytical service, a therapeutic drug monitoring facility, developed. Funding was provided for the development of the Directorate of Linkages and Sponsored Research, of which I shall say more later. The Library received a grant for ICT development. A community oral health project was established in Ife North Local Government Area. Finally, there was a major project, led by the Centre for Gender and Social Policy Studies, to promote gender equity. This included scholarships for female undergraduate and postgraduate students and Fellowships for female academic staff, as well as support for the development of institutional gender equity in the University. These scholarships and fellowships made a major impact on female education in the University. All the projects were successfully executed, largely as a result of the high level of commitment of those involved.

The Carnegie Corporation was prepared to provide two further tranches, depending on how we performed on the first (and second) tranche and on the quality of the subsequent applications. We submitted a second proposal in early 2006, and a second grant of US$2.5 million was approved just before I left office.

The development grants were only a part of the benefits we obtained from the Carnegie Corporation's intervention. The Corporation also funded the training of staff on various aspects of administration and on the development of project proposals, both within the University, with external consultants within Nigeria and overseas. A separate grant was provided for the development of the iLab project, mentioned earlier. The Corporation was particularly interested in promoting advancement activities and sponsored a variety of training programmes in this area. Along with eight other VCs from East and West Africa, I was sponsored on a study tour for VCs in 2003 to examine the funding system in American universities. This was an eye-opener.

American universities receive only a minority of their funds from their governments; most of it comes from advancement and commercial activities and fees. We were able to understand how fundraising activities in these universities were organised and also the roles of university leaders in this activity. It was during this tour that I got to really understand University Advancement. There were differences in how these activities were organised in different institutions. I was particularly impressed by the system in the University of Baltimore, and this influenced my subsequent proposal that we should develop both an Office of Linkages and Sponsored Research and an Advancement Office. The seed of university advancement had been laid. A number of members of staff were sent on advancement training programmes in the

UK and South Africa, and these individuals formed the core of our Advancement team.

I had two trainings. The first one was organised in Abuja in 2003 for the university leaders in the institutions which the Corporation was working with. I attended this with Biodun Adediran, who was the Deputy VC (Academic), and Dele Oye, President of the Alumni Association. I also attended another training in Adelaide during the Commonwealth Universities Conference. These two workshops were very enlightening. We were trained by experts. Two of these trainers made a particular impact on me. They imparted the major principles of Advancement, which I applied subsequently with, I believe, great success. They were Jo Agnew, an Australian, and Lorna Somers, Director of Advancement at McGill University. After I left office, I became a resource person on Advancement courses for CASE (The Council for the Advancement and Support of Education), which organises programmes on behalf of the Carnegie Corporation for African universities. At each course, I would include those principles in my presentations under the title "Useful things I have learnt, mainly from Jo and Lorna, and partly from personal experience." These principles illustrated almost everything that we had done wrong in our early fundraising efforts, including the disastrous Development Fund Appeal. I wish we had received the training earlier.

We knew what we had to do. One important task was to develop a positive image for the University that would make individuals and organisations interested in supporting us, and to develop and cultivate friends and prospective donors for the University. However, we were still encumbered by the image of a university in crisis. Nevertheless, we began to develop friends. We also made the cultivation of good relations with the Press a priority, and I must say that I got on extremely well with the Press. My only problem with the Fourth Estate was that I held rigidly to the principle that press men should not be paid for publicity.

As stated earlier, I paid particular attention to cultivating the Alumni, and I believe my Administration's relationship with them was progressively enhanced. For this reason, we paid particular attention to the Alumni in our fund-raising efforts; these were truly committed "friends" of the University.

The major fundraising success came during the last year of my service. This was the "Renovation Project" to restore the beauty of the University's buildings. The University campus is renowned for its beauty, which comes from its buildings and also from the beauty of its natural environment. Over the years, the horticulture had suffered to some extent, not just because of financial constraints, but also as a result of misplaced priorities, but the deterioration was not severe. I must say that during my tenure we did attend to the problem with some success. The Reforestation Project has been described earlier. On the other hand, the buildings had deteriorated to an alarming extent. None had received even a lick of paint since they were built. Lack of funds has been put forward as the excuse for the failure to maintain these buildings; however, misplaced priorities are also to blame. The buildings looked awful. It was not just the paintwork. Most had flat concrete roofs waterproofed with bitumen felting. The felt had deteriorated and almost every building was leaking. This had to be attended to before any other renovation work could be done. Thus, the first priority was to repair these roofs, and a substantial part of our capital budget each year went into re-felting the roofs, a very expensive matter. What was now required was to carry out the other repairs and re-paint the buildings. There were no funds for this.

I was extremely distressed by the state of the buildings, but gradually a determination built up in me that their beauty should be restored before I left office. One day in May 2005, I mentioned the problem to Wale Adeniran, of Cultural Studies fame. Wale mentioned that the buildings of the Ahmadu Bello University, Zaria, had been renovated with funds raised by its Alumni. There and then, I decided to embark on the Renovation Project, to be financed by funds raised from the University's Alumni. By that time we had not yet established the Advancement Office, so we had to work on an ad hoc basis. After consultations, I set up a committee of individuals who I believed would be committed to the project as well as being knowledgeable about fundraising. These included Professor Tony Adegbulugbe, Professor Funmi Togonu-Bickersteth, Dr. Bimbo Soriyan, Dr. Yemisi Obilade, Dr. Ladi Adeyanju, Chairman of the Home Branch of the Alumni Association, and the Alumni Relations Officer, Lara Adedeji. We agreed that the focus should be on the Alumni; these were the individuals who, having experienced the beauty of the University in the past, would be most likely to support the project. We developed a brochure which described the achievements of the University, both past and present, and its history as Africa's most beautiful campus. The continued beauty of the natural environment was highlighted with photographs, and, finally, the deterioration of the buildings was described. The efforts of the University to renovate some of the buildings were described, again with photographs. By then we had managed to secure funds to renovate Fajuyi Hall and part of the Biological Sciences Buildings. These allowed us to provide "before" and "after" illustrations which also showed that we meant business and could deliver. The brochure ended with an appeal for help in restoring the buildings. The brochure was printed to a high quality and was also available in an electronic form which could be emailed.

I met with the Alumni Executive. By then, Dele Oye's term had ended. His successor, Chief Olu Coker, was also committed to the University. He and his Executive embraced the project wholeheartedly. The branches agreed to hold a series of lunches and dinners to raise funds. The campaign kicked off with a luncheon in the VC's Lodge. We identified individuals with whom we had developed active relationships and I invited each of them personally, emphasising that the gathering was for a select few. The luncheon went very well. The Guest of Honour was Erelu Olusola Obada, the Deputy Governor of Osun State, who had developed a great regard for the University and with whom I had developed a close relationship. The former VC, Wale Omole, also attended and gave a rousing speech in support after I had made a PowerPoint presentation on the project along the lines of the brochure. The participants all pledged support.

Apart from the money raised, Wale Omole pledged to paint the University Hall. He fulfilled that pledge as painters arrived to do the job the following week. The presence of Erelu guaranteed that the occasion, and thus the Renovation Project, received extensive publicity; there was coverage by both TV stations and newspapers.

The Alumni organised eight luncheons, all of which were attended by a team that I led. These were well attended and great enthusiasm was shown for the Project. However, they yielded only modest donations. I realised that the majority of active Alumni were relatively young and so could not contribute much financially. Their major function should be as fundraisers rather than donors, and subsequently we did employ them effectively in that role. The wealthier alumni did not attend Alumni activities, and, more significantly, we had not developed close relationships with them. I must emphasise that one of the principles of fundraising, taught by Jo Agnew and Lorna Somers, was the importance of cultivating prospective donors and involving them in the University before making your "ask." A second was that the alumni are the greatest source of donations (as well as other forms of support) to any university, both as donors and also as fundraisers. One other thing about the wealthy alumni—they tend to move in their own exclusive circles.

Based on these lessons, we modified our approach. We decided to organise dinner parties, hosted by wealthy alumni or friends of the University. These hosts would invite wealthy individuals from within their own circles, and we would supplement this by inviting wealthy alumni whom we considered likely to fit in. There would be a Guest of Honour whose celebrity status would be attractive to the other invitees. The invitations would emphasise the select nature of the occasion, and I personally invited all the guests and interacted with them further before the event. Incidentally, the hosts paid for everything. We held two of these select dinners, both in Lagos. The first was hosted by Dr. Yemi Ogunbiyi, a popular media professional who had been on the academic staff of the University. Wole Soyinka was the Guest of Honour. The second was hosted by Segun and Femi Aina; the first, a businessman with whom we had developed a close relationship, the latter a successful alumnus. Mrs. Cecilia Ibru, the Managing Director of Oceanic Bank at that time, was the Guest of Honour. The guests greatly enjoyed both of the events. During the first, in August 2005, Wole Soyinka mentioned my passion for the University and for the Project. This is another of the principles of successful fundraising—the fundraiser must have a passion for the institution, and be able to communicate that passion to the prospective donor. We raised substantials funds from the two events. One particular donation sticks in my mind; Segun Fagboyegun, a young law alumnus, gave #5 million for the renovation of the Faculty of Law building. He had attended the event because of the regard he had for Professor (Uncle David) Ijalaye, who had taught him in the Faculty. Talk about cultivation!

We supplemented these events with others. We tried to mobilise the University community through meetings and informal interactions, with a varying degree of success. One meeting was with the Deans with the aim of getting them to raise funds for the renovation of their buildings from their own alumni. The then Dean of Science exclaimed that I was now trying to pass the responsibility for renovating the University on to him. In contrast, the Dean of Administration, Professor Kayode Soremekun, went out and obtained the funds with which his Faculty's building was renovated from a multinational company. Nick Igbokwe, Chairman of the Sports Council, renovated the Sports Centre building with funds he obtained from a number of donors. The Dean of Arts, Sola Akinrinade, also took on the idea, and worked with me to raise funds for his faculty. The Librarian raised the funds for the renovation of his buildings. The Students' Union ignored the whole thing. We also succeeded in raising funds or gifts in kind (actual renovations of buildings) from interactions with some individuals and organisations. These included a number of banks. In each of these instances, the donations followed an interaction with a Chief Executive that I or one of my team had gotten to know personally. They were making the donation, not just because they considered the project to be a worthy cause but because they knew, trusted, and had a high regard for the fundraiser. On one occasion, Funmi Togonu-Bickersteth arranged a meeting with Professor Olu Aina in my office. I made my PowerPoint presentation on my PC. There and then, he handed over a cheque for #1 million. I hardly knew this donor, and some would express surprise at such a donation being given under such circumstances, bearing in mind what I have stated earlier about the need to cultivate prospective donors. The fact of the matter is that the donation was possible because Funmi had cultivated the prospective donor. I ostensibly raised the donation, but in actuality it was achieved by Funmi. Incidentally, Funmi Togonu-Bickersteth features repeatedly hereafter, and henceforth she will be referred to as Funmi.

We were able to renovate three-quarters of the buildings in the central campus, as well as Fajuyi Hall, the Health Centre, and a few others. After we had renovated a couple of the buildings in the Staff School, the Parent-Teachers' Association took on the task and renovated the entire school. If others, especially the Deans and the Students' Union, had followed their example as well as those of the Deans of Administration and Arts and the University Librarian, the entire University would have been renovated. The first three major buildings were renovated through contract awards; the staff of the Physical Planning and Development Unit closely supervised them, as I also did. We insisted on a particular brand of paint, to be supplied by the manufacturers, and even got the company to send a representative to train the prospective contractors on its proper application. Subsequently, those buildings that were not directly renovated by donors were renovated by direct labour. In January 2006, Engineer Kayode Adeloye returned from his annual leave. This was an engineer whom I had come to admire for his skills, commitment and innovative ability, as well as his absolute integrity. I asked him to take over the renovation project. He and his small team did a marvellous job. The buildings they took on were repaired and renovated to a commendable standard. They were beautiful. I was particularly struck by the African Studies buildings, whose intricate decorative work was restored to its spectacular splendour. Kayode Adeloye also carried out the task most economically. I estimate that the buildings he handled were done at about half the cost of contracting them out. I remember that Segun Fagboyegun's #5 million renovated not just his old Faculty of Law but also the adjacent Faculty of Social Sciences. I did get Segun's permission to spend the savings in this manner.

A plaque was designed by Steve Folaranmi of the Department of Fine Arts on which we inscribed the names of all the donors and also the names of everyone who had participated in the fundraising and the renovation work. In March 2006, we organised a luncheon party in the VC's Lodge to which we invited all the major donors as well as the project team and the members of staff who had carried out the renovation work. I gave a speech in which I identified each person's role and then we went on a tour of the campus to show the donors what had been achieved with their money. A glorious lunch followed. This is how to thank people. Those donors will certainly give again.

In June 2001, during a discussion on harnessing international support, Wale Akinsola reminded me that the University had on its books a Committee on Relationships with Overseas Institutions. The Committee had not been functioning for many years. The statutory Chairman was the Dean of Arts. At that time, Biodun Adediran was the Dean. I did not know much about him, but I met with him and suggested that he should resuscitate the Committee. It had potential not just to harness international support, but also to attract students and staff to the University from other countries. His efforts were spectacularly successful. We received increasing interest from abroad. A summer programme for students from the United States was initiated in conjunction with Wale Adeniran, based in the Institute of Cultural Studies. Academic grants from abroad began to come in. These were modest beginnings, but nothing had been happening before then. Our overseas connections slowly but gradually expanded. This was when I began to get to know Biodun and to admire his obvious talents in this area. I should add that our friendship gradually blossomed from that time also. Needless to say, I involved Biodun in the Carnegie Corporation development, right from the start. It was he who was actually in charge of developing the successful Carnegie Grant application. When his term as Dean was about to end, I decided that he should continue to be Chairman of the Committee and obtained the approval of Council that the VC should appoint its Chairman rather than that it should be the Dean of Arts. He established a "Linkages Office" to administer the Committee's increasing activities. Influenced by my experiences during the study tour for VCs, we decided to start our advancement activities by formally establishing the Office of Linkages and Sponsored Research as well as a separate Advancement Office, but with the premise that the two, which would have overlapping functions, would work closely together. The Office was approved by the Governing Council in 2003. However, it was pointed out that Senate ought to have been involved in the decision to establish the Office. We took the proposal, actually a fait accompli, to the University Senate but it was repeatedly deferred. There was palpable antagonism to the idea. The Office of Linkages and Sponsored Research has not been approved by the University Senate to this day, but it is one of the University's most effective organs for attracting funds, staff, and students from various parts of the world, particularly the USA.

The subsequent proposal on the Advancement Office, developed by a team under the leadership of the indefatigable Funmi Togonu-Bickersteth, was ready in early 2005. It was to comprise three inter-related units, a Development Office, Alumni Relations, and Communications (Public Relations), with an Executive Director in overall charge. It would operate outside the traditional bureaucratic system of the University and report directly to the VC. We listed it on the agenda for the University Senate, but the paper never got considered. It kept being deferred in favor of "more pressing matters" such as examination results and, of course, the palaver over the withheld salaries. Senate was basically very loyal to ASUU; indeed, many Senate members were more loyal to their Union than they were to the University. Anyway, the paper never got taken. The real problem was actually that there was enormous opposition to the proposal—the age-old conservative position that the Government was responsible for the funding of the Universities and that university staff had no business taking over these responsibilities by getting involved in raising funds held rigidly. In the end, Biodun Adediran and I decided to take the proposal to Council. The paper was taken at the meeting of April 2006. Immediately after I presented the paper, the ASUU members, i.e., all the internal members, protested vigorously, and insisted that the proposal should go to the University Senate first. However, the Chairman, Professor Cookey, stated that this was not necessary and that raising funds for the University was not the direct business of Senate. He went on to give strong support for the proposal. The paper went through. The Advancement Office did not actually take off until after I had left. I did get the physical site prepared. A set of offices on the ground floor of the University was modified and renovated for the Office as part of the Renovation Project.

The Carnegie Corporation gave us a major stimulus on gender issues. In fact, the University had become sensitised to this long before. The Centre for Gender and Social Policy Studies was established in the 1990s and had achieved international recognition. However, within the University, gender equity was largely considered as a theoretical concept from "those in America and Europe." Most male members of the community paid little or no regard to the issue and in effect encouraged women to put home and children before their careers. They also tended to regard them as less capable, such that the science-based disciplines, particularly Technology, were regarded as too difficult for them! The female members of the Community, both staff and students, were so brain-washed by these chauvinist ideas that they tended to fall into line with them, and thus confined themselves to the Humanities. Women were also liable to be promoted less quickly; indeed, some did not have aspirations beyond, say, Senior Lecturer. Very few women in the academic field aspired to, or achieved, administrative positions. The males also tended to look down on women as sexual objects to be exploited; the frequent cases of sexual harassment, exploitation and rape, and how we responded to them as well as the role of WARSHE, have been described in Chapter 21.

I am a committed proponent of gender equity and so were my close colleagues in the Administration. One of my initiatives was a programme of appointments for women as heads of department. Each year I was responsible for making the appointments, based on the recommendations of the deans of faculties. I made it known that I wanted to see women on the lists that they submitted. If a dean's list did not contain some females, I would meet with him and request that this be rectified. The University was actually the better for it administratively; the female heads performed excellently in most cases. I came to regret only one appointment, that of a female lecturer who let her religious biases get in the way of fairness.

Things really got going with the arrival of the Carnegie Corporation, which insisted that gender considerations be built into each of its grants and also included a major grant on Gender in its support. This indeed made a difference. Female staff and students were empowered, not just by the grants but by the realisation of what their rights were and what they were capable of. The gender mainstreaming aspect of the project brought a realisation and an increasing commitment of both male and female members of the Community towards an acceptance of females as equals in abilities, prospects and rights.

The Institute of Agricultural Research and Training (IAR&T) at Moor Plantation in Ibadan is funded by the Federal Ministry of Agriculture but supervised by the University. The VC is the Chairman of its Management Board and the University is responsible for the administration of its personnel. Towards the end of 2002 the Director, Professor J.O. Ojo-Atere came to see me in Ife and informed me that his second term in charge was to end in December. He gave me a list of the senior professors and informed me that it was my responsibility to appoint a new Director. Soon afterwards I started getting anonymous letters making allegations against some of the eligible candidates as well as advancing the causes of some others. I did not know any of the candidates. I asked Professor Ojo-Atere for his advice; he suggested Professor Ebenezer Adebowale. I then asked my trusted friend Wale Adebayo, who, being a professor of Agriculture, knew all of them. He firmly advised me to go with the outgoing Director's advice. I immediately wrote a letter appointing Professor Adebowale as Director of the Institute. It was the right choice. Ebenezer did extremely well. He led the Institute at a time when funds for its primary function, research, had dried up. He established a number of agricultural commercial enterprises, and the profits from this were ploughed into the research activities of the Institute. The IAR&T was one of the few research institutes that functioned effectively during that period. The faithful and very competent Professor Ojo-Atere stayed on in the Institute and took responsibility for some of the enterprises. Two highly capable and very honest individuals; that is all you need to succeed. About three months before Ebenezer's term was to end, scurrilous letters started coming to me once more, and I learnt of unrest in the Institute that was probably instigated by other individuals, including two extremely crooked ones, who wanted the appointment. I immediately issued a letter renewing Ebenezer's appointment, three months earlier than I needed to. The unrest ceased, and so did the letters.

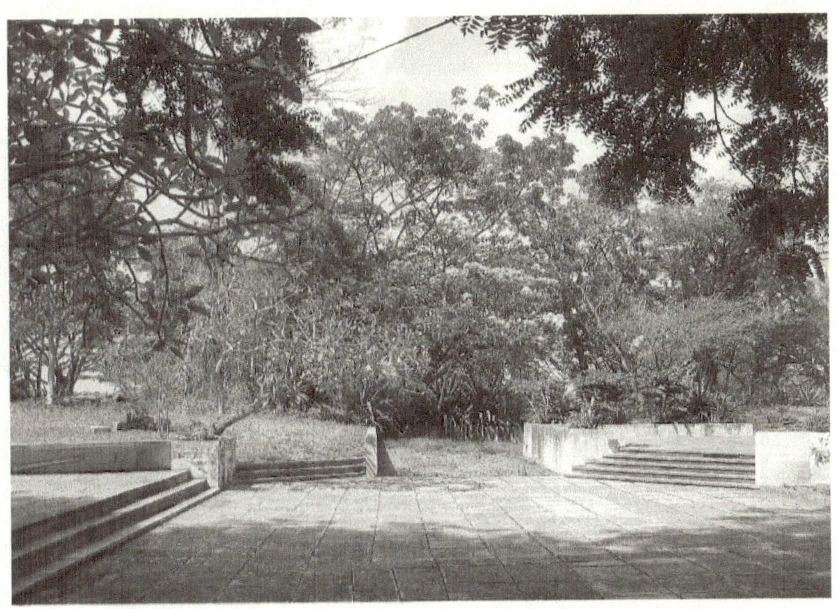

The beautiful gardens in the Vice-Chancellor's Lodge

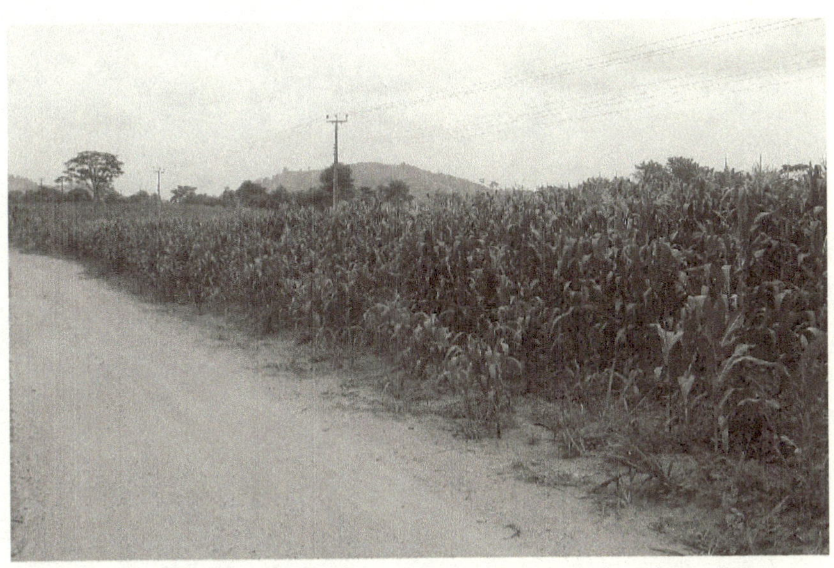

The resuscitated Teaching and Research Farm

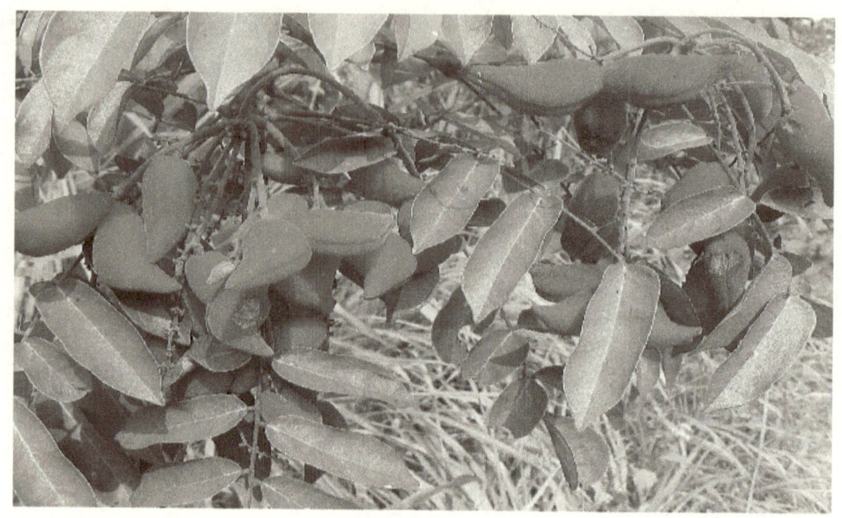

Akara Aje (Cnestis ferruginea), my favourite traditional medicinal plant

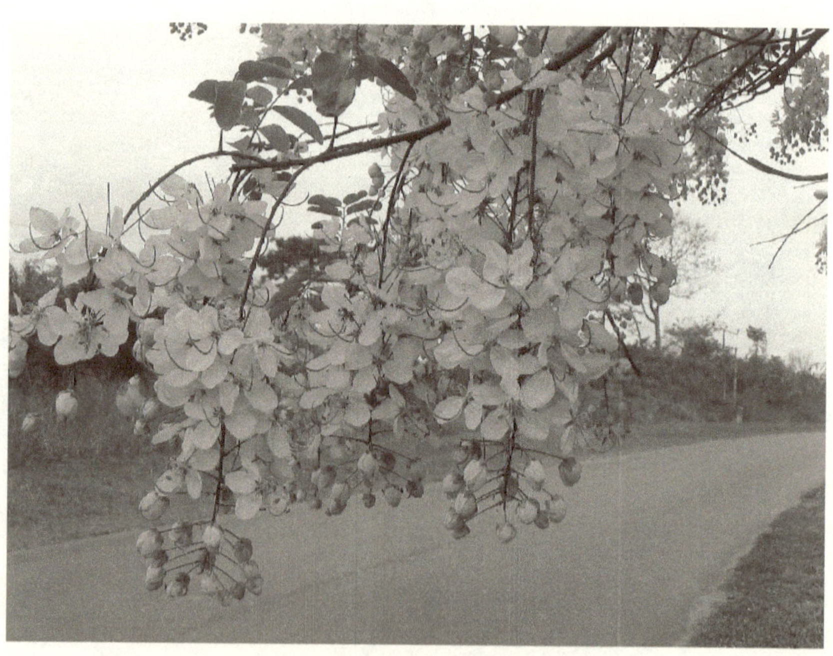

Cassia fistula, close-up

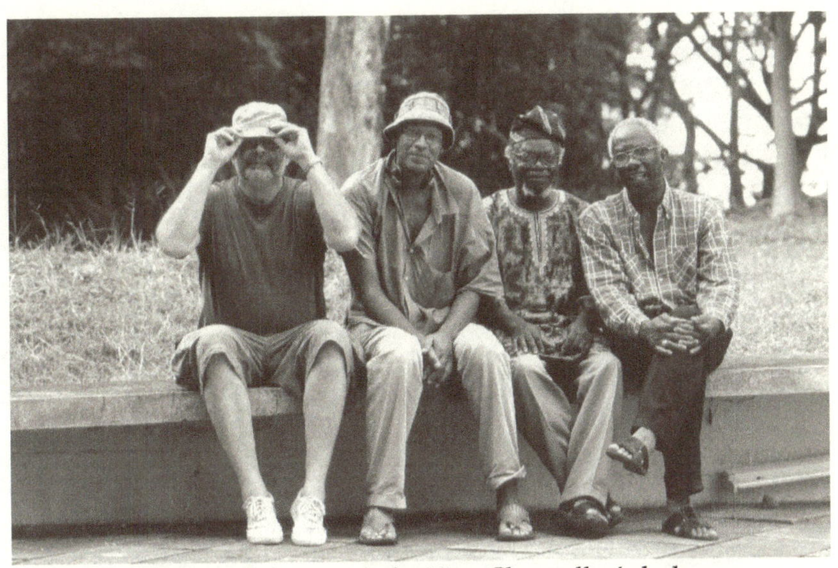

Sunday afternoon at the Vice-Chancellor's lodge
L–R Barry Hallen, Roger Makanjuola, Akin Aboderin and
Lanre Togonu-Bickersteth
(Reproduced with the kind permission of Carla de Benedetti)

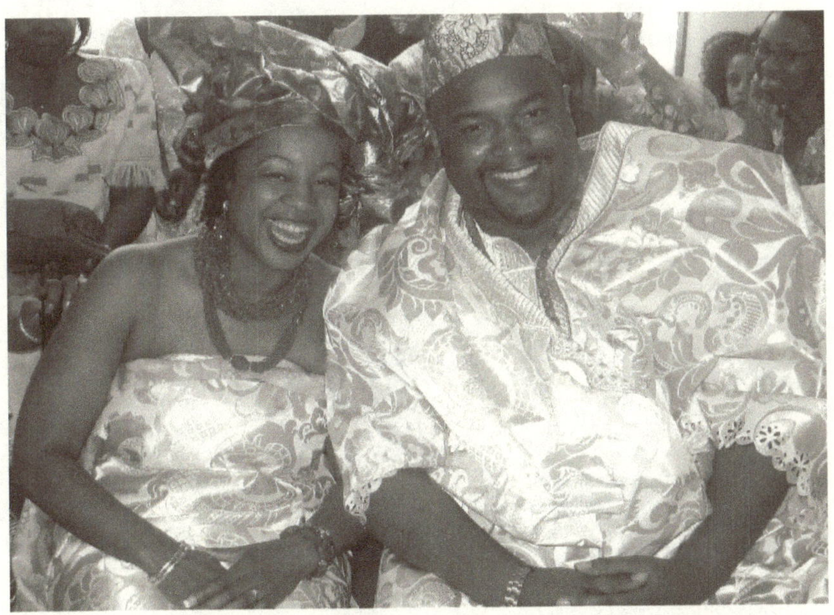

Our children, Nicola and Roger at their traditional wedding

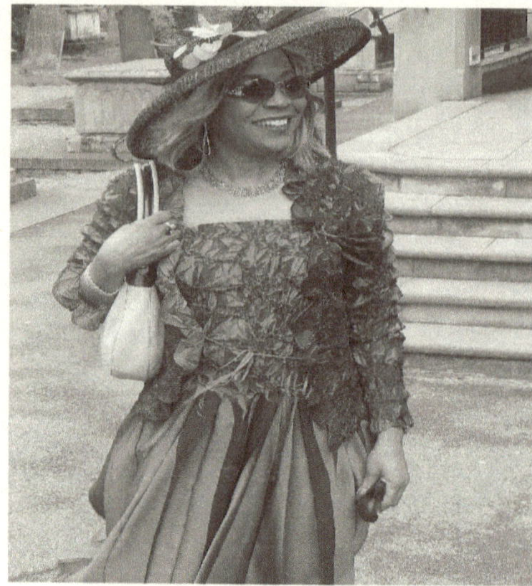

Dorothy at our son
Roger's wedding

Mia, our first
grand daughter

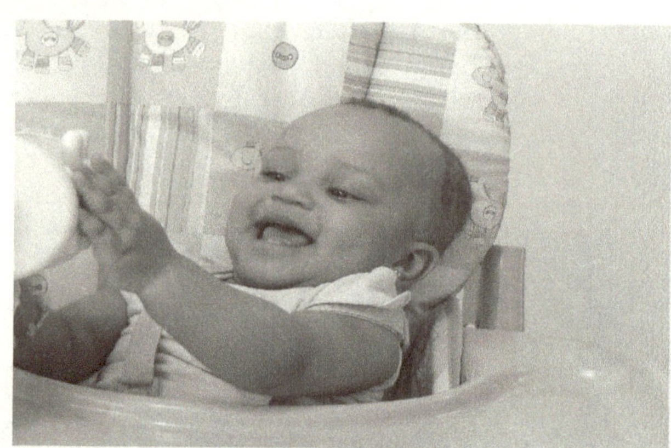

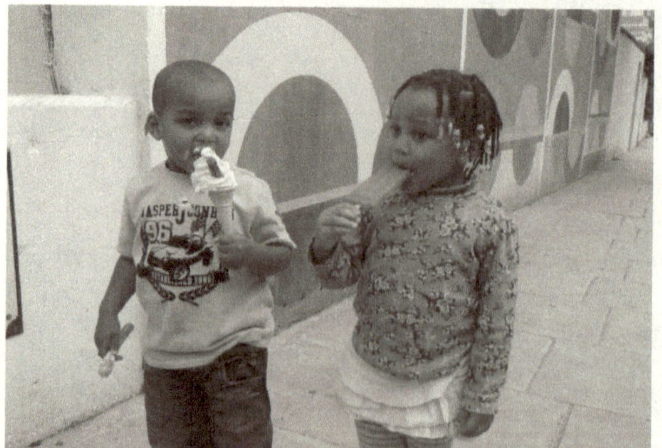

Mekhi and Elena
Makanjuola, 2006

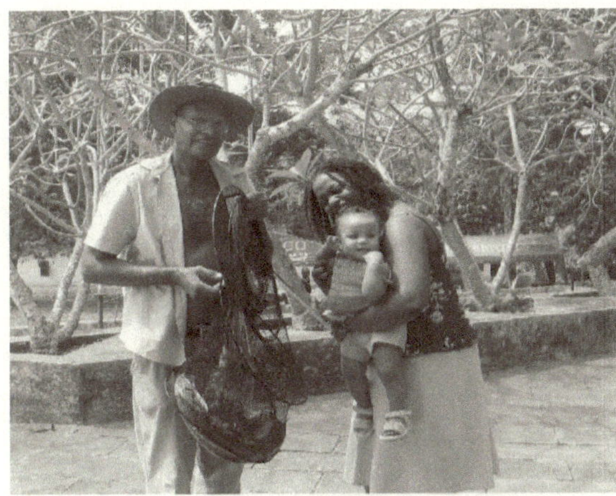

Sunday afternoon—
The Big Catch!
Mia, Wanne and
the author

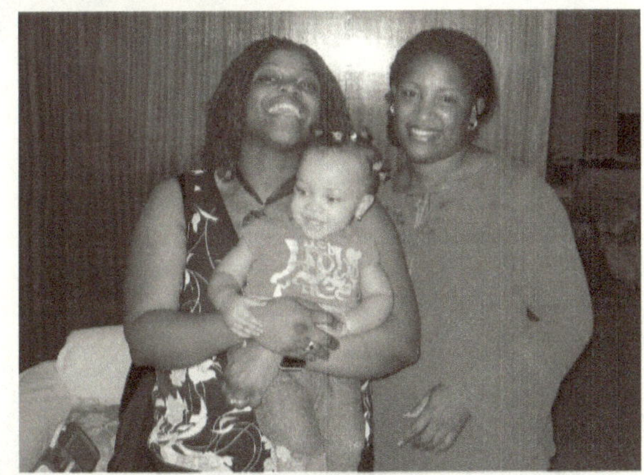

Wanne, Mia, and
friend

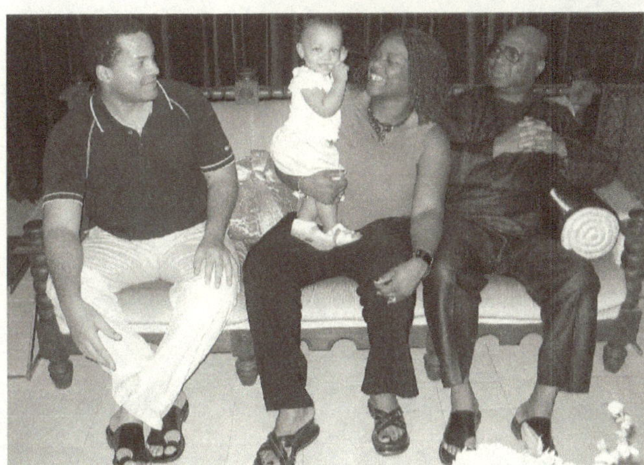

Tony, Mia, Wanne, and Justus, our in-law

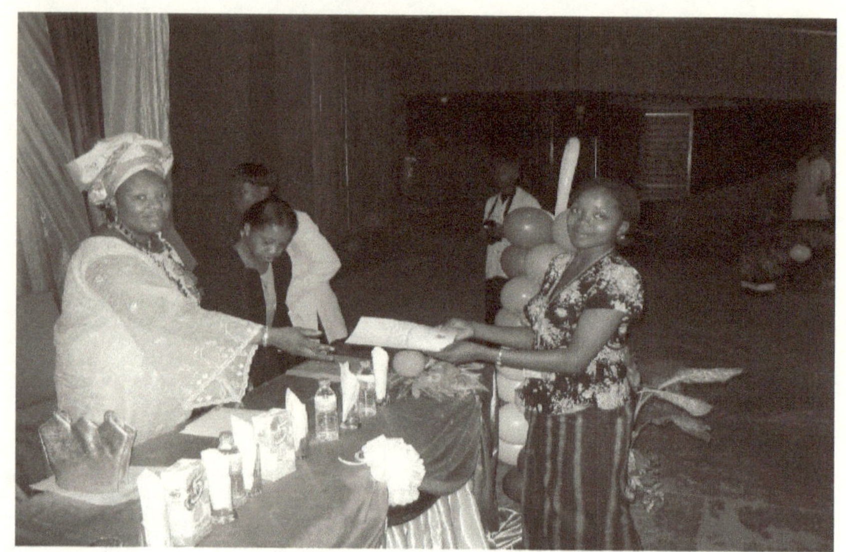

Carnegie corporation female scholarship awards ceremony

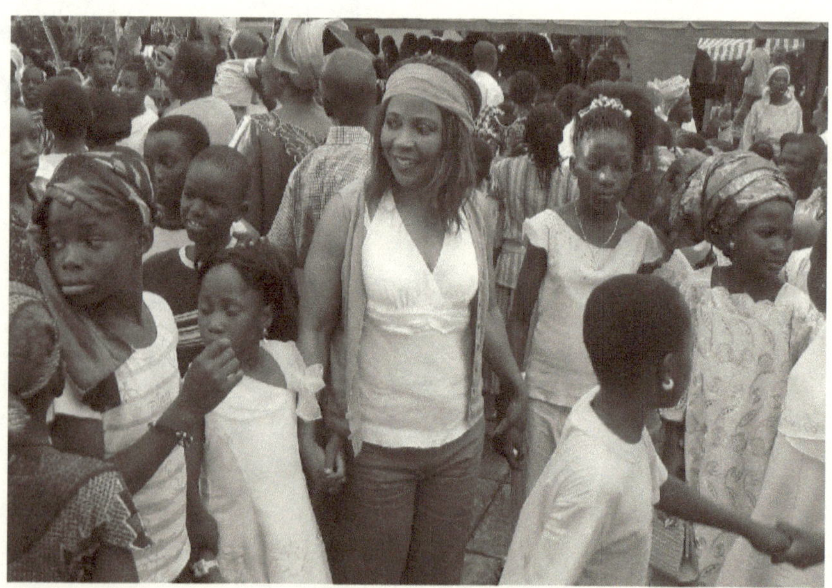

The children's Annual End of Year Party, organised by Dorothy

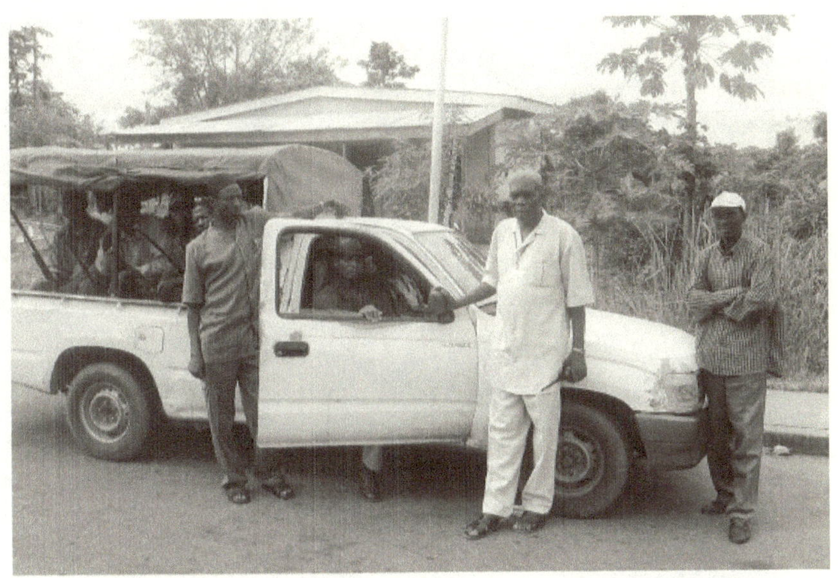

Alhaji Sule Hassan *(second right)* and his Cracker Unit

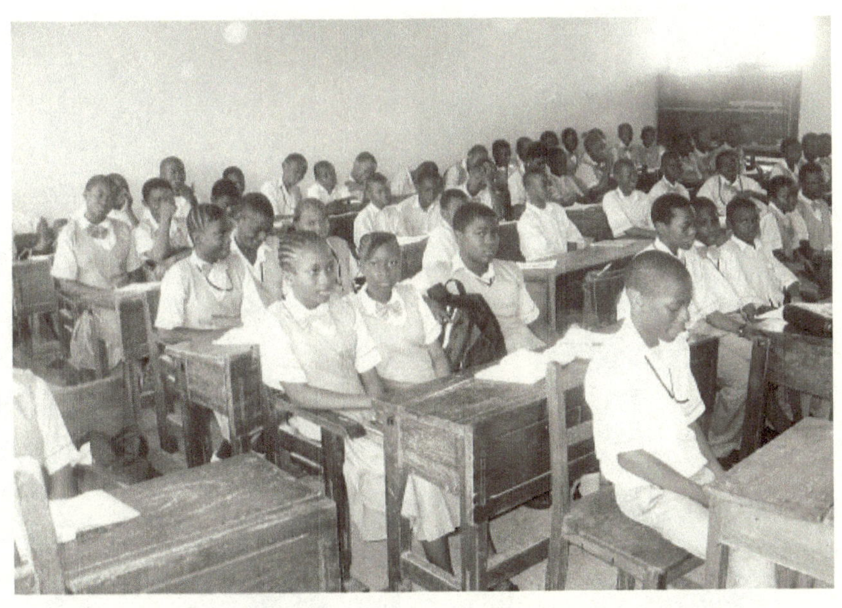

Obafemi Awolowo University International School

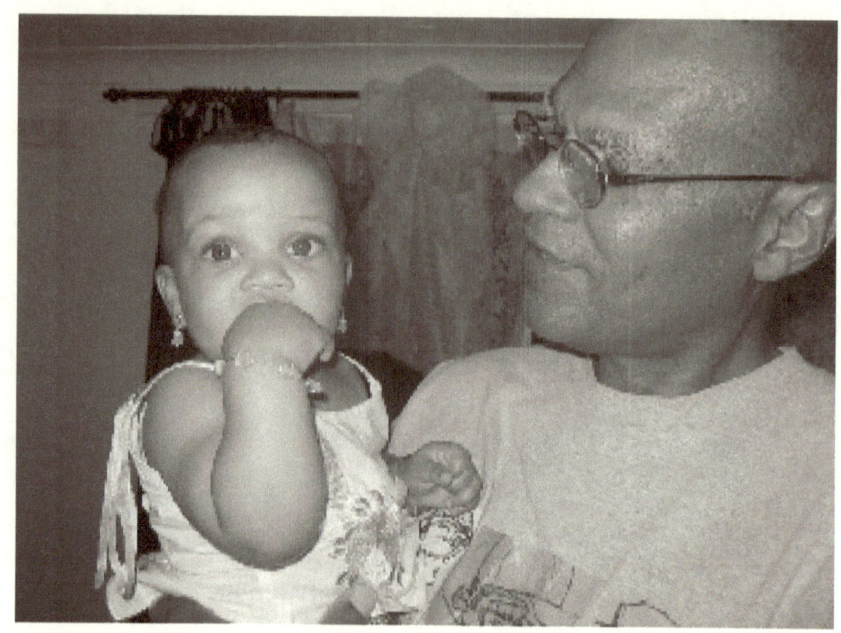

A prospective alumna

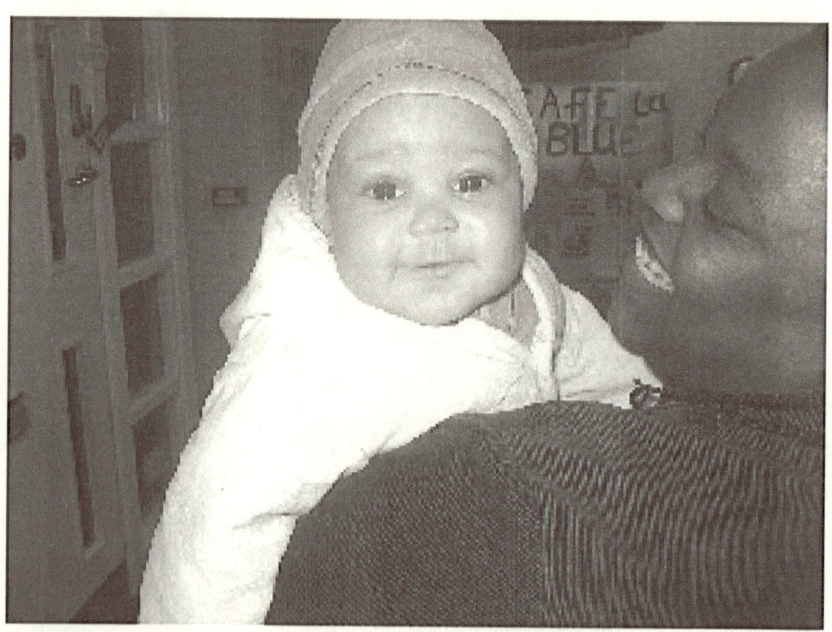

Wanne and Elena Makanjuola: I showed this photograph all over the world — A great fund-raising attraction

XX

The University's Natural Beauty

¤ ¤ ¤ ¤ ¤ ¤ ¤ ¤ ¤ ¤ ¤

The University's land occupies 11, 850 hectares, of which about one-tenth is occupied by the academic area, halls of residence and staff quarters. The Teaching and Research Farm occupies another one-tenth. The rest is forest and bush, dotted with small farms. I have previously dealt with the buildings, and of our efforts to renovate them. The forest and bush land are truly spectacular and very beautiful. The campus is dominated by three large hills on the north-eastern aspect. There is a large reservoir feeding the water works, stretching across most of the eastern aspect. Two smaller reservoirs are located within the Teaching and Research Farm, serving as fish ponds. One of my greatest pleasures is walking through the forest and bush and climbing the hills. "Hill Three," the most eastern, is the highest and most spectacular as well as the most difficult and exhausting to climb. However, the effort is well worth it. From the summit, one can see for many miles, even beyond Ile-Ife city. The vegetation on that hill is also the most varied, both at the top and on the way up. It takes over an hour to get from the Teaching and Research Farm to the final ascent, which is through a natural cave, full of bats. You have to climb up a liana (a climbing plant), which is replaced from time to time when it appears to be getting worn out. I last climbed it over ten years ago, with my sons, Roger and Tony. Since then, I have not been able to find the rather tortuous route and repeated attempts to find it have failed, though I have been able to ascend part of the way. If anyone wants to climb it, there are members of the staff from the Biological Gardens who can show the way. In the past, we used to see a troop of brown monkeys at the summit.

Although I am retired now, I do go back to Ife often. On one of my recent trips, I went for a climb on Hill 2. That climb reminded me to insert a warning about climbing the hills. First, look where you are stepping; if you step on a rock, you may twist or even break your ankle or lose your balance and find yourself careering down the hill, head over heels. The warning applies even more strongly when the ground is wet. I have just had that experience!

As you walk along the paths and climb the hills, you will be absolutely enthralled by the scenery, especially the variety of flora and fauna. Almost every West African bird is present. If you are lucky you will see hawks, or occasionally eagles, swoop down and carry off some small animal. You may flush out a long-tailed nightjar (*Scotornis climacurus*). These are nocturnal birds. They have extensions on their wings so that when they fly, they may appear to be accompanied by two smaller birds on either side—these are the wing extensions. I have never been able to figure out what they are for. There are the beautiful sunbirds. Bushfowl (*Francolinus bicalcaratus*) will suddenly fly off from the ground with raucous calls. Overhead, black kites (*Milvus migrans*) circle in the thermals, looking for the carrion on which they feed; these are among the largest birds you will see. Pigmy kingfishers (*Ispidina picta*), small birds with beautiful aquamarine and orange plumage and large red pointed beaks, perch on a tree or fence, intermittently making their loud cries that sound like a chainsaw—such an ugly call from such a beautiful bird. From time to time they will swoop to catch an insect; these kingfishers no longer fish! Cattle egrets (*Bubulcus ibis*), white birds of the heron family, move around in flocks; on the ground, they move around jerking their heads up and down as they devour insects. My favourite bird is the Senegal Coucal (*Centropus senegalensis*). These are medium-sized birds, with attractive orange-brown plumage on their backs and wings, a white underbelly, and a dark head and tail, which make short but very graceful flights from bush to bush. The Senegal Coucal, called *Elulu* in Yoruba, is said to have magical powers. When it rains, it does not seek shelter, and the Yoruba claim that it brings the rain down on itself and then stays in that rain. Thus, it is an *afowofa* (something which brings trouble upon itself). If one suffers from a problem or illness that one has brought upon oneself, for example through drug abuse or offending a deity or ancestor, this bird may be used in the antidote. There are two varieties of hornbill common on the campus, the Allied Hornbill (*Lophoceros semifasciatus*) and the Grey Hornbill (*Lophoceros nasutus*). Both are medium-sized birds, distinctive for their large curved bills and dipping flight. The Grey Hornbill is actually grey brown on its dorsal surface and near white on its underbelly. The Allied variety has a stippled brown dorsal surface and a grey underbelly.

On the three reservoirs, there is additional birdlife. The most plentiful are a variety of water fowl. I initially thought these were ducks; however, they have longer necks, and stand with their heads raised rather than retracted. They also have narrower beaks. I identified them from a manuscript by Reverend Father Farmer, titled Birds of the University of Ife Campus, as a variety of grebe. I once shot one and it was prepared in *Oga* Arigbabu's house as pepper soup. It tasted awful. There are two types of heron, a smaller white one and a larger grey one. These spend most of their time standing in the shallows, absolutely still, with sudden strikes with their long beaks at passing fish. Kingfishers also abound, mainly pigmy kingfishers. You would think these would take the opportunity of proximity to the water to catch fish. They do dive into the water, repeatedly, but still only to catch insects on the surface, as do those we see in the gardens. On the main reservoir, there used to be a pair of kestrels. I have not seen them for over 15 years. Lily trotters (*Actophilornis africanus*), birds with red bodies, white throats and dark crowns and with long gangly legs, run on top of the water as though always in a panic. On the main reservoir, you will also see some beautiful black and white birds that spend most of their time standing on the platform above the water intake, with occasional brief flights. I have not been able to identify them. Finally, swarms of small, dark-brown birds fly around repeatedly diving onto the surface of the water. I have not identified them either, but they are a nuisance to fishermen. We often mistake the ripples they make on the water from their dives as the ripples from surfacing fish. I have mentioned only a few of the birds. There is an abundant variety of birds on the campus. Almost every bird listed in J.H. Elgood's book Birds of the West African Town and Garden are to be found there. Father Farmer's book The Birds of the University of Ife campus is also a useful reference, especially for the water birds, which are not listed in Elgood's book; however, it lacks the former's beautiful illustrations. The campus is full of birdsong. This starts at about 4am, reduces during the heat of the day, and builds up again as the day gets cooler. The sweetest of these birdsongs, to me, at least, comes not from the nightingale family, which are not represented on the campus, but from the prolonged musical call of a bird that I have not been able to identify for certain but which is most probably the Red Eyed Turtle Dove *(Streptopelia semitorquata)*.

Apart from the birds, the animal life is profuse. Rainbow lizards are probably the most common of the reptiles. On the hills and rocks they are largely replaced by skinks, smaller lizards with brightly coloured tails. There are two types of squirrels. The tree squirrels are the most abundant. They occasionally set up house in the roofs of houses. We had a family of them in our former house on Road 11, until one day the house was invaded by soldier ants. These ants, known as *Ijalo* by the Yoruba, certainly live up to their reputation that nothing can stand in their path, except kerosene and insecticide!. The squirrels escaped en masse, squealing in agony. The house was also swept clear of cockroaches on that occasion. The ground squirrels or *ikun* are larger and are frequently seen crossing roads or paths from one stretch of bush to another. Various varieties of rodents are flushed out as you move around. The largest of these, the grasscutter or *oya (Thryonomys swinderianus)*, are greatly prized as bush meat. The meat is certainly delicious; however, I stopped eating it after I discovered that the *oya* is no more than a giant rat. The Etu, Maxwell's Duiker *(Philantomba maxwellii)*, a small brown antelope, is said to be not quite as delicious, but I personally find it much more acceptable on the dinner table. The largest animal on the Campus is the Igala, a truly beautiful antelope that may reach the size of a small cow. It is an attractive orange-brown colour, with white flecks. It is extremely graceful in its bounding flight. On one hunting expedition, two igalas were flushed out but subsequently disappeared. Aided by beaters, we tried to find them. Suddenly, the two came out from behind me, obviously very frightened, but they looked so beautiful that I could not fire. Actually, although I have been on a number of hunting expeditions, I have never shot anything! My pleasure on these expeditions comes from walking around with the hunters through the bush and seeing the animals. Most of the mammals are nocturnal and thus in daylight they will only be seen if they are flushed out. However, their tracks abound on the bush paths and farms.

As expected, snakes are plentiful on the campus. They are everywhere, and sometimes come into houses. Some huge pythons have been reported, including some claimed to be large enough to swallow a human being. Most of these stories are probably exaggerated. Most snakes are fairly small. The majority of West African snakes, up to 85% of them, are non-poisonous. The most common poisonous snakes are the Green Mamba, found mainly on trees, the Gaboon viper *(Oka)*, and a number of varieties of cobra *(Sebe)*. The problem is, that you can never tell which snake is poisonous and which is not unless you are an accomplished expert who can recognise a snake from its shape and colouring. Most often the proof of danger lies in looking into their mouth to see if there are fangs! Most people are not prepared to go that far! So we tend to kill first and, perhaps, ask questions afterwards. One important piece of advice—when in the bush, always look where you are stepping. Also if you are overcome by the need to do a "number two" in the bush, make sure the area is clear first – there is one variety of cobra which is particularly prone to biting unsuspecting individuals squatting to do it where the snake is resting. Scorpions most often live under rocks. They may be driven out by rain, and another source of danger from them is if you get tired and decide to sit on a rock that houses them. We all fear scorpions. However, a bite from one of them is rarely, if ever, fatal, though extremely painful.

The bats—Ife is famous for them. They were estimated at over a million on the campus in the 1980s. These are the African Straw Coloured Fruit Bat (*Eidolon helvum*). They spend the day hanging from very high trees, in large clumps. They are a truly remarkable sight at dusk, when they start their nightly journey to find food. As their name implies, their sole diet consists of fruit. Why they have to travel such large distances when fruit is available all over the campus remains a mystery. They are also migratory. At the beginning of the dry season they disappear, presumably to greener pastures, and return at the beginning of the rainy season. In the 1990s, they disappeared from the campus, presumably because of being excessively hunted. However, in late 2000 they returned. I mentioned their reappearance in my manifesto, stating that "even the bats are back," with the implication that my period as Acting VC had attracted their return! However, it soon became clear that they were a mixed blessing. They stopped their annual migration, presumably because their safe habitat had been progressively destroyed. Thus we had increasing numbers in continuous residence on the campus. There were so many of them on each tree that the branches would collapse. As a result, many trees, particularly oil palms, were destroyed, and the canopies of the more sturdy trees were distorted. We eventually had no choice but to begin to disperse them, much to the chagrin of Professor Eyo Okon, a world renowned authority on these animals. We sent the Cracker Unit out regularly to shoot them. During these expeditions, we were treated to another truly remarkable sight. Each shot was immediately followed by a mass flight of the bats, totally obscuring the sun and bringing temporary darkness. Only a few would be killed during these expeditions. Repeated shots and the smell of gun smoke, which the bats do not like, would make them vacate the campus. Unfortunately, before the trees recovered they would return. With the increasing destruction of their natural habitat, tall trees, they found the campus a relatively safe environment, at least until the Crackers went after them again. Incidentally, they are greatly prized for their meat. There was a ready market for them; the proceeds of the bat hunts went to the purchase of ammunition for the Crackers. For those who may be somewhat apprehensive about coming near them, these are fruit bats, they do not bite. They do carry a virus, the Lagos Bat Virus, which infects animals and not humans.

Almost every specie of West African plant is found in abundance on the campus. Although the activities of the failed sawmill and poachers reduced the number of economic trees, the forests are still luxuriant. One tree that I searched for and could not find was the *Yohimbini* tree (*Pausyntalia yohimbe*). This is known as *barantashi* by the Hausa, who use its bark to make a potent male virility drug. The active ingredient is *yohimbine*, a virility agent that preceded Viagra. I understand that the West African forests have been denuded of this plant as a result of over-exploitation. The Re-forestation Project has been looking for samples for propagation. The trees on the University blossom at the end of the dry season and the early rains and at that time the campus is truly beautiful. *Cassia fistula* is probably the most beautiful. This produces a swathe of yellow flowers which resemble large candelabras. Road 2, in particular, is a long line of yellow when they are in bloom. There are also three large ones on the main road leading into the campus and which appear in marvellous succession as you drive into the University, and many more on the edge of the "Motion Ground" in front of Oduduwa Hall. The Jacaranda blooms for much longer and has luxuriant bright purple flowers. There were many of these trees on the campus initially. However, their trunks tend to break easily during rain storms, so they have gradually been reduced in numbers, some through storm damage, but more through being felled as a precautionary measure. Several have been felled unnecessarily. One problem I observed was that residents on the campus felt threatened by any tree on their grounds and tended to want them felled. It is true that some species are relatively fragile, but most are not. I issued a directive that no tree should be felled without my express permission, and when a request came through, I usually inspected the tree myself. I usually refused permission, to the annoyance of the applicants. But have you ever heard of an *Iroko* or an *Ogano* tree falling down? In some cases, the residents felt so strongly that they would still go ahead and use whatever means they had at their disposal to fell the tree, since the Parks and Gardens Unit would refuse to carry out the task. One senior lecturer, having been denied permission to fell an Iroko tree in his garden, denuded the tree of its bark. The tree died and fell on his house in the night. The house was destroyed. He denied responsibility and claimed that the tree had been damaged by some *Orisa* worshippers!. We moved him to a guest house, which caught fire soon afterwards, when he left the house during a power cut without turning off the electric cooker. This man must have been jinxed.

The end of the dry season is signalled by the blooming of the flamboyant, Flame of the Forest, trees. As you walk down bush paths, you suddenly come across the bright red canopy of this tree—nothing could be more beautiful. It truly deserves its botanical name of *Delonix regia*.

There are fruit trees in every compound, and also on the roadsides and in the bush—mangoes, guava, and every possible variety of citrus; you name it, we have it. As I walked around, I would occasionally help myself. There is nothing more delicious than a mango straight from the tree. I operated on the theory that although the tree belonged to the house's occupant, the fruit hanging over the fence was community property! There is a fascinating array of shrubs and smaller plants on the hills and bush. In the 1980s, I carried out a research project on traditional medicinal plants. Most of my specimens were obtained from the Iwo area, which is a transitional zone between savannah and rain forest, and thus a good source of plants from both zones.

One Saturday, I spent two hours tramping through the bush along with my guide, Mr. Olanihun, looking for a plant called *Akara Aje*. I returned to Ife triumphant, with this plant and some other specimens. The following day, while fishing on the bank of the main reservoir, I looked behind me to see that plant growing in abundance on the sandy soil. *Akara Aje* (*Cnestis ferruginea*), is so-called because of its bright red fruit. In Yoruba folklore, red is the colour of the *Aje*, which is the Yoruba equivalent of the European witch. Thus, where *Aje* is believed to be involved in the causation of an illness or other misfortune, this plant may be employed in the remedy. It is my favourite medicinal plant.

Another enthralling experience is the view of the sky at night. When there is no moon (and particularly so when there is no electricity!), the view of the stars and planets is truly spectacular. The first to appear, and the brightest, is the planet Venus, arising from the west and gradually travelling eastward during the course of the night. Mars and Jupiter are also easy to see, most times of the year. The constellations and the Milky Way are all beautifully displayed. The easiest to identify is Orion, with its three-starred belt and nebula beneath. The Pole Star is usually easily identifiable at the end of the Little Dipper.

Of course, things were not perfect. The Parks and Gardens Unit was under-staffed. More importantly, the Unit was very short of equipment, and what was available was largely obsolete. Thus, much of the work of maintaining the grounds was done by hand, with cutlasses and hoes. I did give priority to the needs of the Unit, but practical (financial) considerations placed a limit on this. Nevertheless, the Unit performed well under the circumstances, although when the rains were in full flood, some areas tended to become overgrown. Mr. Jacob Abuah was the Head of the Unit initially, and was a very competent horticulturist. He was the only professional initially. Under pressure from a member of academic staff who wanted me to employ his wife and kept harassing me over it, I de-froze a position of horticulturist. We interviewed applicants for the position along with interviews for the position of water engineer. I was very particular about getting a competent individual for the post of water engineer, so I chaired the interviews myself. As I mentioned, we had created the position for the lecturer's wife. However, another candidate, Mrs. Lolade Oyedapo, performed much better, and we had to employ her, much to the chagrin of the lecturer. Mrs. Oyedapo was a relatively junior horticulturist; however, she turned out to be extremely competent. Her commitment is illustrated by the fact that two days after she gave birth to her first child (we did not know she was pregnant!), she came to work on an Okada (commercial) motorcycle! She took over as Head of the Unit when Jacob Abuah retired.

On reflection, we did not deal with environmental miscreants firmly enough. We were very firm on the issue of farming in inappropriate sites; those who did not abide by the rules, for example, farming in front gardens or on the roadside, had those farms destroyed. However, there was an even worse source of environmental pollution—illegal structures comprising shacks and makeshift garages and stores which constituted a real eyesore. We should also have dealt with these.

Incidentally, the interview at which we appointed Mrs. Oyedapo also yielded a really good young engineer for the Water Engineering Unit, Ayo Oyeniran. He performed far better than the other candidates, and to cap it all, he is an alumnus of the University. He had a good basic knowledge of his profession, came across as honest and, above all, was willing to learn. In spite of his relative youth and junior status (the then Acting Head of the Water Engineering Unit was on a higher grade level), I insisted that he should move into the office of the Head of the Unit. The former Acting Head, a technician, tried to sabotage the arrangement. He declined to show him how the system worked and engaged in subtle antagonism, so I sent him on an extended leave. Kayode Adeloye and I put him through the operations of the water supply system. He learnt easily and became a true asset. He was devoted to the work. During one period of problems with the water supply and when the students were up in arms, I got worried one night over possible sabotage and drove to the water works at 4am. I found him there, personally running the system. I never had to worry about the water supply after that; I knew I could depend on him.

Garbage was another major problem. The Health Services had old refuse lorries and tractors that kept breaking down. We kept repairing them, but we really should have procured new and more advanced refuse disposal equipment. On reflection, one of my major errors was in not finding the funds to buy new equipment for the refuse disposal system, including modern refuse trucks. Refuse collection was often irregular, both to the halls of residence and the staff quarters. The problem in the staff quarters was aggravated by the attitude of the staff. Shamefully, many did not have dustbins, and even when we procured some, they refused to buy them. Some of them, including at least one professor, would dump rubbish at the back of their gardens. Others would dump the rubbish on the road. A PhD is not necessarily an indication of true education.

My life was fairly stereotyped; you could easily predict where I would be and what I would be doing at any time. My working week began early on Monday and ended in the early afternoon on Saturday. I tried to keep the rest of Saturday and the whole of Sunday free, though this was not always possible because of emergencies or official commitments. I would drive to work in the Pajero at around 7am. I did not eat breakfast except on Sundays, and started the day with two cups of tea and one of coffee in the office. My first task would be to clear emails before the official working day started. Thereafter, the time would be filled with meetings, inspections of projects, and other commitments. "Lunch" consisted of snacks such as *akara*. I went through the mail towards the end of the day, after the other staff had gone home, and would then drive home at around 7pm. When I got home at night, I would eat a large supper, watch TV for a while, and go to bed around 9pm. On Saturdays, things were more leisurely. I would get to the office around 9 am and work till 1 or 2pm.

The VC's Lodge is a beautiful white building, constructed during the time of Professor Hezekiah Oluwasanmi, who is widely credited with most of the work of developing the

University. He was a truly great man, and only posthumously acknowledged as the real builder of the University. The Library is named after him. In my opinion, this is not adequate recognition of his contribution. There are four bedrooms and a small TV room upstairs. The ground floor consists of reception and dining areas and a study. The Lodge contained two beautiful artefacts. The main entrance door was of *iroko* wood, carved with images depicting traditional royal scenes. There was also a reproduction of Ben Enwonwu's "The Rising Spirit" in the main hall. In the 1980s, a "born again" VC decided that these two beautiful items were fetish and had them removed. I found the door in the garage and the statue in the boys' quarters, along with another carving. I restored all of them to their place.

I was on my own for most of the time, and in fact only used one bedroom, the TV room, and the kitchen. I used to do the major cooking of stews and so forth at weekends, and the steward would cook the rice or whatever accompaniment I wanted each night. The stewards and I ate the same food. I wonder what they thought of my cooking! Whenever Dorothy came over, she would stock the freezer with stews, vegetable soups, and so on, so I would not have to cook for some time thereafter. Initially, I had three stewards and a laundryman as well as Grace Odere helping in the house. For some months after the strike action of September 2002, when all of them deserted me except Grace, I kept her alone with me. Following Dorothy's subsequent intervention, I kept two stewards, Laurence Oyeyemi and Mudasiru Raji. I did not retain the laundryman and later transferred him to the Health Centre where his services were much more useful. Grace did the washing of the laundry and I ironed it. On reflection, I lived as a recluse; not really the expected thing of a VC. However, I did have to modify this lifestyle periodically when work demanded that I entertain guests. On such occasions, I would pull out all the stops, for example when the Alumni were in town or during fundraising events.

I looked forward to my weekends. On Friday night, I would stop at the Staff Club, where we had an outdoors area that came to be known as the "Elders' Corner." Here I would share a few beers with my friends in a relaxed atmosphere. Even my detractors in ASUU would share this friendly atmosphere with the notable exception of Otas Ukponmwan, who on a number of occasions subjected me to loud and very strong abuse in the Club. On Saturday evenings I would go for a walk and climb through the bush and the hills.

Sunday was the most pleasurable day. After the early morning service at All Souls Chapel, I would have breakfast and then go fishing with *Oga* Arigbabu and sometimes also other friends who fished more occasionally. We fished with rod and line. In the early days, I employed mainly floating tackle, whereby the baited hook was presented to the fish from a float on the surface, weighted down with a piece of lead between the float and the hook. Bites are detected by the movement of the float as the fish tugs on the bait. When a bite is detected, the hook is, hopefully, embedded in the fish's mouth by a sharp upward movement of the rod, termed a "strike." You then reel in the fish. In recent years, we have tended to use the technique of legering more often, although I still occasionally bait a floating tackle with a small fish for pike, that most vicious of predator fish. With legering, the float is dispensed with, and the baited hook is cast to the required spot and kept on the bottom of the water by a lead weight. Bites from fish are detected by movement of the rod tip or slackening or tightening of the line. If the rod is held in the hand with the line kept reasonably taut, then the bite can actually be felt through the rod. The tackle we use—rods, reels, lines, and hooks—used to be available in Nigeria or Togo; now it has to be purchased from abroad. We make weights ourselves from casting molten lead from old car batteries, and floats can be made using corks from wine bottles. If you cannot afford the imported tackle, which is quite expensive, £50–£100 for a good set, then you can use the local technique of a raphia pole, twine, hook, and float made from a piece of calabash or other gourd. However, this local rig has very limited range and you often have to enter the water to get in range of the fish. This is not advisable because schistosomiasis is rampant in Nigerian fresh waters, and some waters contain leeches. The most common fish of any size are the *tilapia*. There are three major species, *Tilapia zillii,* dark in colour and which develops deep red colouring when breeding, *Tilapia galilea,* which is more silvery in colour, and *Tilapia nilotica,* the Pink or Giant *Tilapia,* which earns these two names from the pink tinge on its undersurface and its tendency to grow to a large size. "Pinks" are also the most delicious. *Tilapia zilii* and "Pinks" are most commonly caught during those periods in the dry season when they move inshore to breed. They stay around the sites where they lay their eggs, and because they cannot forage for food, they are more likely to go for your bait. The normal diet of *tilapia* is *algae,* and, for this reason, they are more likely to be found around sunken logs or other vegetable matter. The best bait for them is a variety of large worms that are found in the soil around river banks. If you do catch a "Pink," please look into its mouth. These fish carry their eggs, and subsequently, their young, in their mouths whenever they sense danger. If you do see eggs or their young, please put the fish back in the water.

Catfish (*Clarias* spp.) are less commonly caught, except on the smaller of the reservoirs on the Teaching and Research Farm, which is stocked with them. These are ugly, dirty looking, scaleless fish that may grow to an enormous size. They are foragers, and swim along the bottom swallowing anything that attracts them, so you can catch them with a variety of bait. I believe small fish or pieces of fish are best, but they will also go for large worms. The biggest fish that I have caught, on the main reservoir, weighed two and a half kilos—eight of us ate it. The largest I have hooked was much larger than that. This was in 2009 when I was casting with worms in front of the spillway of the main reservoir. I felt a violent tug, struck, and hooked this monster. I battled with it for over 20 minutes. First, it dragged my line out about 100 metres and I could not reel it in; it was that powerful, I had to gradually release the line, while maintaining the pressure. It then came in towards the shore and entered a clump of raphia. My line was stuck there and I decided to wait, knowing that it would move eventually and perhaps get loose again. After five minutes it did move out again, and I found that my line was no longer stuck in the raphia. The fight continued. The fish was tiring, and I was able to gradually reel it in using the technique of "pumping." This involves raising the rod tip to pull the fish in, then lowering it and reeling in the slack so produced on the line. A long and laborious process, but if you just try to reel in, the reel will not turn easily and is likely to be damaged. Gradually I brought the fish in towards me, and at last I could see the monster! It was tired and no longer struggling. As I lifted it out of the water, the line broke under its weight and it swam off. If I had had a landing net with me, this would not have happened. After a repeat of the experience, possibly involving the same fish, a week later, I started going to the spillway with a landing net. Unfortunately, I never hooked such a large fish again. I cannot say for certain how big the fish was—my guess that it was somewhere between seven and ten kilos. The line that broke had a 12lb (5 kg) breaking strain. I no longer eat catfish; its dirty appearance and thick covering of protective slime have put me off. I catch them frequently, and give them away.

Occasionally, we hook the Elephant Trunk Fish, (*Mormyrus rume*) on the main reservoir. These are so-called because their snouts are long and curved downward like an elephant's trunk. These fish, called *Osan* by the Yoruba, are reputedly delicious, and are a particular specialty of restaurants in the Republic of Benin. They move around scooping up rubbish from the river bed and sieving this out through their gills, so they are caught with a rod and line only by accident, when they suck up the hook with other debris as they swim around. Finally, there is the African pike (*Hepsetus odoe*). These are elongated, vicious looking predators that normally feed on small fish. Thus, they are best caught with small fish as bait, but will go for a worm also. They are ferocious fighters, and will put up a great fight after they are hooked. They have a fearsome set of teeth; indeed the lower jaw has two rows of these sharp, pointed teeth. As you are reeling in, they have the habit of jumping out of the water and cutting the line. We try to get round this by using a tracer, a length of wire, between the hook and the line, but often they will still get away by jumping out of the water and cutting the line above the tracer. Pike are very bony, and not as tasty as catfish or *tilapia*. Nevertheless, the excitement of catching these ferocious predators makes up for that. Our Sunday morning expeditions would start with digging for bait on the banks of the reservoir or its streams. The fishing itself would last for between one and three hours, depending on whether we were catching fish or not. We would exchange a variety of jokes, mostly of a scurrilous nature. Exhausted, we would return to the VC's Lodge with our catch, and then the real fun would begin. I had a small circle of friends, who would congregate at the Lodge for the afternoon. Apart from *Oga* Arigbabu, there were Biodun Adediran, Kwashi Ako-Nai, Wale Adebayo, Juliet Dixon, Sumbo Abiose, and, occasionally, Bayo and Dolapo Amole and Akin Aboderin. Sumbo, whom I have not mentioned before, is a Food Scientist and has been a family friend for many years. Akin Aboderin is a retired Professor of Biochemistry who now lives in Ibadan but comes to Ife regularly. I have two other friends, Barry Hallen and his wife Carla de Benetti, who also featured prominently whenever they were in the country. Barry used to lecture in Ife but now works in the United States. Carla is an internationally renowned photographer. We would sit in the shade in the beautiful gardens of the Lodge, consuming copious quantities of beer and wine. If we had caught any fish, pepper soup would be prepared. There was always *suya*, bought the previous day in the Staff Club and microwaved. When Dorothy was around, there were more substantial offerings; she is a great cook. We relaxed in the gardens, surrounded by frangipani, flamboyant, and *Bohemia gmelina* trees. The latter blooms with abundant, delicate pink flowers. The happy and relaxed atmosphere was well and truly captured by a photograph of four of us taken by Carla, which is in my sitting room wall in London. The conversation would range from developments in the University, through politics and, of course, scandal. We could discuss any subject, secure in the trust we had for one another. Nothing we said ever went beyond this small, intimate circle of friends. The group has continued even after I left office. We are envied. Many would like to join, but we have kept the circle exclusive. We trust each other.

I have gone to great lengths to show the beauty of the flora and fauna in our Ife campus that most people never see, nor explore during their stay in the University. The administration and crises in Ife challenged all of us, but its beauty sustained and particularly reinvigorated me. I have travelled the world over, and I am yet to find a campus more beautiful than Ife. Ife is where my heart is and where I always return to with joy.

XXI

Relationships

During my years as an administrator, I met many people; some had a positive influence while others had a negative influence on my life. Whether good or bad, these people remain in my memory and this chapter is dedicated to them.

I worked with four Federal Ministers during my term as Chief Medical Director. Professor Olikoye Ransome-Kuti appointed me though I hardly knew him. Over the next four years, I got to know him very well and I believe he was convinced about my commitment to the institution and to patient care. He went as far as declaring his confidence in my integrity in the pages of the newspapers some time after my tenure ended. Olikoye Ransome-Kuti was one of the finest individuals that I have ever known. Olikoye was the eldest of three brothers. Next to him was, Fela, a world-renowned musician; the youngest, Beko was a medical doctor. All three were in the forefront of the fight for human rights and social justice in the country. They all stood firm against corruption, which Fela defined and called "authority stealing" in one of his songs. Corruption has for many years been the bane of Nigeria. I used to quote from Fela's song Authority Stealing during lectures on Administration.

> *"Armed Robber him get gun,*
> *Authority man him get pen,*
> *Pen get power gun no get.*
> *Armed robber, him go steal 80 thousand naira,*
> *Authority man him go steal 12 billion naira,*
> *You no go hear them shout, thief, thief, thief..."*

Beko was a true hero of the Nigerian people's fight for democracy and justice.Olikoye was a paediatrician, but through most of his career, he actually functioned as a community physician. In his early professional years, he realised that most of the illnesses afflicting Nigerians were preventable or easily alleviated by early diagnosis and treatment which could be met effectively through a robust primary health care system. He spent the greater part of his professional life promoting primary health care as the essential base of the health care system. When, in 1985, General Ibrahim Babangida appointed him Federal Minister of Health, his chance came to implement his beliefs. He developed Nigeria's National Health Policy which is still in operation today, providing for a firm base of primary health care, supported by suitably developed secondary and tertiary (specialist) facilities. This system of health care has been adopted all over the world. Most people will remember him for that. However, there was much more to him. He was a true example of the dedicated physician, renowned for his commitment to the care of his patients and for his compassion towards them. When he was in charge of the children's emergency ward of the Lagos University Teaching Hospital (LUTH) in the 1960s, mothers, knowing that he would always show up in the early hours of the morning for a ward round, would waylay him in the corridors of LUTH at 6am to seek his help for their children. He always willingly attended to them. There was no time for strikes in his day.

As Minister of Health, Olikoye demonstrated the three values that are, to my mind, most important to mankind—hard work, honesty, and honour. These are values that, unfortunately, no longer have much credence in Nigerian society. This was a Minister who arrived at work at 7am. If I needed to see him urgently, I would waylay him in his office at that time, knowing I would always find him there, and he always attended to me. He was absolutely incorruptible. He never took a kobo from anyone, he despised corrupt people. He vehemently accused some African governments of stealing donated funds targeted for medical care. In 2001, he told a WHO conference that only $12 out of every $100 contributed by donors eventually got to HIV patients in most African countries. At one international conference, he publicly stated, "I have seen 300 million dollar presidential palaces and $350 million cathedrals in the midst of ill-health, poverty, and destitution in various African countries." Perhaps I should add one further quality—his humanity. He really cared for people.

Professor Olikoye Ransome-Kuti influenced my life the most over the last quarter of a century. He was always ready to support my efforts, to give me advice and encouragement. He was a shining example to me. I wanted to be like him. I was truly delighted that my University awarded him an honorary doctorate degree, although it ended up being conferred posthumouly.

In preparation for the hand-over to civilian rule, the appointments of all the Federal Ministers were terminated in 1992. Prince Julius Adeluyi was appointed Secretary for Health. He was there for only a short period, and the interim nature of the Government meant that significant activity was at a minimum. Nevertheless, I got on quite well with him. Dr. David Tafida was appointed Minister under the Abacha regime. He was extremely knowledgeable and committed. I found him to be straightforward and very supportive. However, he did not last long. Abacha reshuffled his Cabinet after only a year or so.

For most of the Abacha years, from 1995 to 1997, Chief Ihechukwu Madubuike was the Honourable Minister. I was at first quite impressed by him. He appeared to be motivated by a wish to transform the health care system, and he held a number of meetings with Chief Medical Directors during which he appeared to appreciate what the problems were and what needed to be done. When he decided to organise a "National Health Summit", I believed it was a genuine attempt to critically evaluate the system and develop realistic solutions. I enthusiastically participated in the event and presented two position papers. The summit cost several million Naira. Chief Madubuike claimed that a new National Health Policy had been produced from the recommendations of the summit, but this has never seen the light of day.

In 1996, we felt that we were ready at Ife to carry out a kidney transplant. To this effect, we needed a new haemodialysis machine to back up the transplant service. At that time, we did not have a Board of Management, and the Ministry of Health was responsible for approving contract awards. I went to Chief Madubuike in Abuja and requested that the contract be urgently approved. We had the required funds. He told me to submit the relevant documents to him and that the approval would be processed immediately. I submitted the documents and waited confidently for the approval. When after one month I had not heard anything, I went back to him. He directed me to a "Projects Office" which he had set up and through which it appeared that all contracts were being awarded. I found that the documents were lying in that office and receiving no attention whatsoever. I was made to understand that "negotiations" were required concerning which company should be awarded the contract. I left and wrote the Minister a letter expressing my disappointment. Other CMDs gave equally harrowing tales. Contracts for the supply of specialised equipment such as haemodialysis machines could not be awarded to just any company.

Navy Captain Anthony Udofia was the Military Administrator of Osun State between 1993 and 1996. The institution got into his good books when a truck full of Air Force men had a serious accident on the Ife–Ibadan road. Many died, and the injured were brought to the Ife Unit. I returned from a trip to Lagos and stopped over in the hospital at about 7pm to find the Accidents and Emergencies Department very busy. Seriously injured airmen were everywhere and they were so many that some were being treated on the floor. I initially joined in the emergency efforts. However, after a few minutes, I began to think more clearly and started mobilising the various specialty teams that were required; mainly surgery and dentistry. The response was instant and marvellous. Everyone that was contacted came to the scene immediately regardless of whether they were on call or not. An important element of emergency care in the hospital was the provision we had introduced, that everything required should be provided in emergency cases, whether the patient could pay or not, so the materials needed were readily provided. The operating theatres were in use all night. Many lives were saved. I felt really proud of the hospital and of our efforts, as we all did.

The Chief of Air Staff came to the Hospital the following weekend, accompanied by Navy Captain Udofia and a team of officers. They were extremely impressed with our efforts. The Chief of Air Staff had come with a substantial amount of money. I told him not to pay anything then and that we would send him the bill. He could not believe it! Navy Captain Udofia later told me that because of the way we had handled the casualties, as far as he was concerned, I could "do no wrong"! This high regard and goodwill stood us in good stead subsequently. Whenever I visited him he always received me with the greatest courtesy. During fuel crises, he would send fuel tankers to us. He also helped me once over a personal problem.

The Ooni of Ife, Oba Okunade Sijuwade Olubuse II, has featured both in my account of my time in the Hospital and in my period as VC. I wish to emphasise here that he gave me great support throughout. I was welcome in the Palace any day; he would receive me immediately and dispensed with formality. He called me *Omo Oba* because my uncle was the Oba of Imesi Ile. There was no reasonable request that I made that was not met. Once he gave an undertaking, no follow-up was required. He believed we were making a major difference to the care we were providing for the Ife people and stated this at every opportunity. When the hospital decided to organise a second phase launching of the OAUTHC Development Fund Appeal in August 1992, he persuaded Chief Sonny Odogwu to be the Chief Launcher, General Yakubu Gowon to be the Chairman and the Emir of Kano to be the Chief Guest of Honour. The occasion attracted many dignitaries. Apart from these three individuals, we also had Alhaji Shehu Shagari, the former Head of State, Mrs. Victoria Gowon, the Governors of Oyo and Osun states, and the Chief Justice of the Federation. The publicity was tremendous. However, the event yielded only a little over one million naira, or 50% more than we had spent in organising the event! I have since learnt much more about successful fundraising. The Kabiyesi was so impressed with the performance of the hospital that he conferred an honorary chieftaincy on Dr Abiola-Oshodi.

The other major traditional ruler in the Ife-Ijesha area is the Owa Obokun of Ijesaland, Oba Adekunle Aromolaran. In the early period of my administration as CMD, he complained bitterly about how the institution had run down the services of the Wesley Guild Hospital which had been taken over from the Methodist Mission in the 1970s. He eventually expressed appreciation for some of the developments we implemented in Ilesa, but he never really gave us much support. Much later, when I visited him as Vice-Chancellor of the University, he criticised my administration. Apparently, he had received negative reports about us from some people, and he launched into open criticism without even bothering to hear my side of the story. However, in Ilesa, we did have some great supporters. Outstanding among them was late Chief Lawrence Omole, probably the most prominent of all the Ijesa businessmen. He was a delightful person, a man of great dignity, extremely courteous, open and very friendly. He supported us in everything we wanted to do for the institution. At a time when most of the Ijesa people, including the Owa, were busy criticising us, he financed a borehole for the Wesley Guild Hospital. Unfortunately, the yield from the borehole was inadequate. He was truly delighted when we finally executed the Ilesa water project. Lawrence Omole's philanthropy extended beyond the hospital. He had been extremely supportive of the University in its early days, and was rewarded with an honorary doctorate. His senior wife, Mrs. Moni Omole, was one of the founding members of the Baby Friendly Initiative in the hospital. She was also an extremely kind, pleasant, courteous person; her whole demeanour was of goodness.

Many years ago, in a private conversation with Professor (Uncle) David Ijalaye and the late Professor Arthur Okunniga, I stated that "All politicians are thieves." Both vehemently made one correction to that statement. They insisted that there was one politician who had never stolen a kobo—Chief Adekunle Ajasin. Chief Ajasin was the foremost politician in Ondo State. He had worked side-by-side with Chief Obafemi Awolowo. He served as Governor of Ondo State from 1979 to 1983. I first met him through his wife, the dignified, delightful, and compassionate Mrs. Babafunke Ajasin. She had consulted me over a minor medical problem which had been easily resolved. Chief Ajasin himself later developed medical problems and I was contacted. I mobilised consultants from the hospital to visit him in his home in Owo. We were initially able to treat him. Sometime in 1995, Chief Ajasin was brutally confronted and subjected to verbal assault in his own home by the then Military Administrator of Ondo State. His medical condition was exacerbated by the incident, but subsequently improved. Chief Ajasin had a cardiac pacemaker that had been inserted in the United Kingdom. When the pacemaker failed, he was brought to our hospital. However, we did not have the facilities to deal with that problem at that time, so he was transferred to the UCH, Ibadan, where a new pacemaker was inserted by Professor Wole Adebo. A few weeks later, Chief Ajasin suffered a fracture. He was then staying in Lagos, but insisted that he be brought back to Ife. I was very proud. Dr. (now Professor) Lawrence Oginni successfully operated on the fracture. Chief Ajasin recovered once more and returned to Owo. A few weeks later, he suffered further problems and was brought back to Ife, where he died in our Intensive Care Unit on 3 October 1997. There was a strike action by junior staff in the hospital at the time and, aided by two medical students, I had to carry his body down to the mortuary of the Ife State Hospital, where Chief Ajasin's body was embalmed. I then personally drove the body to our newly commissioned mortuary at the Wesley Guild

Hospital in an ambulance. Over the period of his illness, I got to know Chief Ajasin fairly well, and developed a tremendous respect for him. Chief Ajasin combined my treasured values of honesty, hard work, and honour with humility, so being one among a handful of individuals to whom I have been able to ascribe these values.

Dr. Babalola Borishade was the Special Adviser to the President on Education in July 1999. After the 10 July murders, it was he who advised President Obasanjo and the Minister of Education to appoint me as Acting VC. He is an alumnus of the University and was on the academic staff until 1989, when he resigned as a Reader to enter the private sector. Oddly enough, I hardly knew him, but he had clearly been keeping in close touch with events in the University and also knew of my performance in the Hospital. He gave me excellent advice in those early days. He succeeded Professor Tunde Adeniran as the Federal Minister of Education in February 2001. For reasons that are not clear to me, ASUU had developed a strong dislike of him and organised a campaign to prevent his being appointed Minister. In fact, they succeeded at first, since his appointment was initially rejected by the Senate. The campaign continued, and eventually he was shifted to Aviation.

Much has already been written about his predecessor, the extremely pleasant Minister, Tunde Adeniran, who was so supportive.

Professor Fabian Osuji followed in August 2003. He was quite a contrast to the other two. He was one of the most arrogant individuals I have ever met. Whenever I managed to get into his office to see him, he would sit at his desk without a hint of courtesy, snobbishly addressing me as "Makanjuola" during the interaction. Although we did not get on well, I felt much sympathy for the manner in which he was booted out of office. He was accused, along with a number of senior officers in the Ministry, of bribing National Assembly members to approve a favourable budget for his Ministry. There has been public insinuations and outcry that Ministries distribute largesse to National Assembly members in order to ensure a generous budgetry allocation. As far as I know, the charges against Professor Fabian Osuji were quashed by the Court of Appeal Abuja Division.

Chief Bisi Akande was the Governor of Osun State when I started. He is one of the few politicians for whom I have admiration. He was remarkably honest and very open in his administration. He is a very principled person. He was very supportive of me and the University, but the support was largely moral. I believe he had a high regard for me, probably because he believed I was honest too.

Prince Olagunsoye Oyinlola took over in 2003. He is an alumnus of the University, but I believe the reasons for his support of the University went beyond that. He gave us great support. I have mentioned earlier his role in the Fortieth Anniversary Development Fund Appeal. There was no time we asked for his help that we did not receive it. I was even able to get a donation for the West African College of Physicians when we had our Annual Meeting in Nigeria. In 2005, I visited him and requested for a bus. At that time, the State Government was donating buses that were labelled *Oyin ni, o,* a play on his name. This means "It is honey, o." I told him, "We too want an *oyin ni, o!*" He smiled and approved it. He approved a number of grants and other support to the University. He was very concerned about the 2003 crisis and intervened, though his efforts were unsuccessful. When his Government approached us with a proposal for an agricultural project, I received this very enthusiastically. This was our opportunity to give something back, and I made personal efforts to ensure the success of the project, chairing most of the planning meetings. I even benefited personally from his goodwill after I had left office. When the State Government executed a road project in Parakin Estate in Ile-Ife, I discovered that the roadworks ended just before my site on the estate. I took a letter to Prince Oyinlola, requesting that the work be extended to include my site. There and then, he authorised it; we are talking here about a cost of a million naira or more.

Prince Oyinlola's deputy was Erelu Olusola Obada, a lawyer. I first met her in 2003, when she came to chair a seminar on campus. At that time the lifts in the University Hall were not working. I met her downstairs and then we both had to climb the seven floors to my office. She had great difficulty doing this, and we had to stop several times. She was not pleased at all, and I had forebodings of a difficult relationship. However, during the ceremony we got along well, and over the next three years, we developed a good relationship, and she also became well disposed to the University. I found her to be extremely articulate and highly intelligent. She was by no means a token appointee; she had major responsibilities in the State Government which she faced with great commitment and ability. She is a very warm, very charming person. Finally, she is beautiful! Just like the Governor, she supported the University tremendously. She was extremely generous to us.

The National Universities Commission (NUC) has a supervisory role over the University system, although its powers have varied over the years. I worked with two Executive Secretaries. When I started my tenure as Acting VC in July 1999, Professor Munzali Jibril was the Executive Secretary. He was a very pleasant, quite humble individual. He was always instantly accessible and I found him to be very supportive. In September 1999, he provided a "loan" of ₦50 million when I informed him that we could not pay salaries for that month. He said he would deduct the money from future subventions, but he never did. During the communal crisis of 2000, he got the NUC to approve ₦8.4 million to construct a hostel block; the only proviso was that the building should be named after Chief Simeon Adebo, the former chairman of the NUC. When he was not granted a second term as Executive Secretary, I was quite disappointed, and felt, as he did, that he had been hard done by; he had been doing a good job. Professor Peter Okebukola was appointed in August 2001. He was younger than Munzali, and had innovative ideas, directed at modernising the University system. He gave major priority to the promotion of modern technology, especially ICT. He had great ideas, and he embarked on the promotion and development of ICT in the NUC and within the University system. I must say that some of his ideas may not have been adequately planned. This applies particularly to the "Virtual Library" based in the NUC, on which there was major investment but limited success. He initiated a number of moves to improve the funding of the universities, and used his political acumen and relationships with the Presidency and within the National Assembly to get them approved. The budgetary allocations improved somewhat, and he also got the approval for a "Direct Teaching and Laboratory Costs" grant, which was made available to departments and had a major impact on teaching. He was very pleasant and I liked him a lot. He gave me a lot of help. During the crisis of 2003 he gave the University a loan of ₦100 million to pay the salaries of those who were at work. Subsequently, he found a formula whereby the loan did not need to be repaid. Our problems probably started in 2005, when he learnt that we had paid the withheld salaries to the staff. I confirmed that we had paid the salaries and that this was because I was fearful for the very existence of the University. He appeared to accept the explanation and even came across as sympathetic. However, I later learnt otherwise; both he and President Obasanjo were determined that the "No work, no pay" principle should be upheld.

My real problem with Peter Okebukola, which I must accept was a personal one, came after the accreditation exercise for university programmes that took place in 2005. We had prepared extensively for the exercise. We held meeting after meeting with Deans and Heads of Department and attended to all the deficiencies we could identify. Where there were shortages, we hastily recruited the required academic staff. The physical facilities were repaired; fortunately the Renovation Project had started. I had to attend the Annual Meeting of the West African College of Physicians the week before the visitations, but flew back early to attend to any last minute problems and to inspect our physical facilities. I met with the cleaning contractors for the academic areas and gained their cooperation to ensure that the campus was in pristine condition. The visits took place over a two-week period. We met with each team and I had the impression that things were going well. I was absolutely flabbergasted when, some weeks after the visits, Professor Okebukola phoned me to say that our Law programme was to be denied accreditation. I had been away when the visitation team for Law had given its feedback, but Biodun Adediran, who met with them, confirmed that the team had made negative comments. I found it difficult to believe, because just a couple of months earlier, the Council for Legal Education had made a visitation to the University and been so impressed with our facilities that they had increased the number of students that we were authorised to admit each year from 150 to 250. Three days after the Executive Secretary had phoned me, I went to the Governor's Office in Osogbo to take delivery of the donated bus. The media men were there and I took the opportunity to brief them on developments in the University. During the interaction, one of them asked for my reactions to the loss of accreditation for our Law programme. The results had been published, but I had not yet seen them. I responded that, if this was true, the loss of our accreditation in Law was totally unjustified. We were proud of our Law programme and its facilities and would immediately take steps to get our accreditation restored. In the heat of the moment, I probably was quite assertive in stating my position. My comments were widely publicised in the newspapers. Professor Okebukola phoned me and stated that the NUC Management had held a meeting over the publications and that he was going to make a strong statement to the Press concerning my comments. The next day, he held a press conference in which he stated, "The VC is posturing like a student who has failed an examination and refuses to accept the result." I was extremely offended by those remarks. In retrospect, the Law programme did have deficiencies. We did not have enough senior academics and our library collection was inadequate; it was full of antiquated volumes. When the Chairman of the NUC, Chief A. Ayimonche, herself an alumna of our Law Faculty, visited the University at my invitation, she met with the Faculty and also visited the Law Library. She unequivocally confirmed the deficiencies. This was a committed alumna, with whom I got on quite well. I believe her assessment was correct. We immediately began on measures to rectify the deficiencies. A year later, the Law programme was granted interim accreditation; by then I had left office. I am happy to report that full accreditation was restored in 2009.

I first met Chief Oyekunle Alex-Duduyemi in the early 1980s, when he was the chief donor to a Lions Club project that I was involved in. He was always ready to help the University, and we exploited his generous nature repeatedly while I was VC. This quiet wealthy man is one of the most cultured Nigerians that I have ever met. He has a fabulous residence on the way in to Ife, with a large lake stocked with fish that grew to enormous size because they were left alone. *Oga* Arigbabu and I went fishing there a number of times. On each occasion, even if he was absent, the steward would bring us an ice-cold bottle of champagne.

Soon after I resumed office as VC, the Chancellor, Alhaji Umaru Ndayako, the Etsu Nupe of Nupe, resigned—I never met him. In February 2001, the Emir of Katsina, Alhaji Kabir Usman, was appointed Chancellor. This was a truly delightful man, a gentle, kind individual with whom I got on well. Each year, the Pro-Chancellor and I would visit him in his palace to formally invite him to the Convocation ceremonies. It took two days to get there, with a stopover in Abuja. We would be received formally, with the Emir, then in his late 70s, surrounded by a retinue of senior advisers and his colourfully dressed Dogari. The discussion would last no more than 15 minutes, and then we would be off. A two-day journey for a 15-minute meeting! This was the tradition. Nevertheless, we were obviously greatly honoured by the courtesy and the kindness with which we were received. The Emir would travel to Ife for the Convocation Ceremonies with a huge retinue. Well, I thought it was huge— about 10 senior advisers and 20 Dogari. However, I have been told that some Chancellors of other universities travelled with even larger retinues. Throughout the period of Convocation, he conducted affairs with great dignity. One problem we had was that he would not shake the female graduands by the hand. The tradition in Ife is that each graduand will come forward and receive a handshake from the Chancellor. On the first occasion, he shook hands with the males, but when the females approached, he would clasp his hands together and bow to them. In fact, by this behavior he was showing the ladies proper respect. His religion, Islam, did not allow physical contact between a man and a lady who was not his wife (or, I presume, his daughter). On that first occasion, I got up and shook the hands of the females. Subsequently, we decided that I should shake the hands of all the graduands while they bowed to the Emir. When I was going to introduce my wife, Dorothy, to the Emir, I warned her not to shake his hand. She curtsied to him, and was about to back off when he seized her by the hands and received her as though she was his daughter. We both felt greatly honoured by this kindness. He showed me much affection and was extremely upset by the events of 3 November 2004. The Emir died in March 2008 after a brief illness. I was greatly saddened. Incidentally, his son succeeded him as Emir and also as Chancellor of Ife.

The Principal Officers, who were essentially my colleagues in the central administration of the University, were myself, the two Deputy VCs (Academic and Administration), the Registrar, the University Librarian and the Bursar. In addition, we worked closely with the Chairman of the Committee of Deans, and we included him in most major decisions. We had an ad hoc "University Management Committee" comprising these individuals which met monthly as well as when there was a particular need, usually some crisis or the other. At the height of its antagonism towards me, the ASUU executive complained that the Committee was illegal, because there was no provision for it in the University Statutes. However, I have never come across any organisation that does not have such arrangements.

The efforts of Professor Wale Akinsola have been described earlier. He was my first Deputy VC (Academic), and we worked together very effectively. He is very capable and we achieved much. He led the development of our Strategic Plan and showed great acumen in supervising the complex administrative set-up in the University. He also had a flair for political issues, something that I never mastered. He was a good administrator.

Although we got on well, we did not have a particularly close relationship. Initially, I worked without a Deputy VC (Administration), carrying out the duties of that office myself. After a year, I decided to look around for a suitable candidate. I found one in Professor Lawrence Kehinde of the Department of Electronic and Electrical Engineering, who had earlier been appointed the Director of our ICT set-up, the Information and Communication Technology Unit (INTECU). I felt he was very capable, and I also knew him to be absolutely honest. I approached him in September 2001. He was initially lukewarm, and I asked him to think about it; the University, of which he was an alumnus, needed him. After a month of further interactions, he agreed, stating that he had prayed over the matter, and had received a positive response from his God. I had to put up a second candidate; no way was I going to repeat the stupid error I made when the Deputy VC (Academic) was appointed. I persuaded Professor Augustine Isichei to stand. At the Senate meeting on 3 October 2001, Lawrence was elected by a large majority. He served as Deputy VC (Administration) for four years (two terms). Lawrence carried out his duties admirably. The job largely concerns supervising the support services of the University—power, water supply, health and environmental services and maintenance. He had a good understanding, indeed a good knowledge of these areas, and the interpersonal skills to motivate those involved. During a strike action by NASU and SSANU in September 2002, he learnt how to run the power house (I was the tutor!), and we shared that burden. He combined his duties with directing INTECU; he did that job equally effectively. He was absolutely trustworthy and very loyal. Lawrence and his charming wife are committed Christians; he is actually a pastor. Thus our interests were somewhat disparate, and, although we got on well, we were not as close as I became to subsequent Deputy VCs.

When Wale Akinsola's term was due to expire, I approached Biodun Adediran, whom I had placed in charge of the Committee on Relationships with Overseas Institutions, the predecessor of the Linkages Office. He readily agreed, and was elected at the Senate meeting of 13 August 2003. When Lawrence's second term expired, I opted for Professor Bayo Amole as a replacement. Bayo is a close friend and was closely involved in the planning and supervision of capital projects in the University in his joint capacity of Chairman of the Projects Advisory and Project Implementation committees. He remains a true friend, and I have described in an earlier chapter the episode of, "Roger, how can I help?" after the University Senate had more or less condemned my actions during a strike action by NASU, as well as his subsequent organisation of the water tanker services. His wife, Dolapo, is also a delightful person and so are their two boys. I put up Kwashi Ako-Nai, the Director of the Central Science Laboratory, as the second candidate. I regarded both as being highly competent to do the job, but I had actually wanted Bayo Amole to be elected. Kwashi won. I suspect that Senate knew I was closer to Bayo, and this was at the height of my unpopularity with the academic staff. However, I was still pleased; I knew Kwashi could do the job, and I trusted him. The period when I worked with these two Deputy VCs was a very happy one for me. These were two highly committed individuals who were well suited, indeed, ideally suited, for the two tasks. Both were well liked by the community and this made up to some extent for my own unpopularity with the academic staff. Biodun, in particular, was an astute politician. He understood the social dynamics of the University Community and had the diplomatic qualities that I lacked. He was thus invaluable in soothing ruffled feathers during crises or in anticipation of trouble or whenever I had trod on people's toes. Above all, we trusted each other implicitly and supported each other. There is nothing worse than having to look behind your back because you are not sure about what your colleagues are doing. This was never the case with Biodun and Kwashi. We became very close friends; we shared similar interests and our personalities complemented one another. We remain extremely close friends to this day.

Mrs. Bola Iluyomade was the Registrar for most of my period in office. She was a very experienced and highly capable professional who had risen through the ranks of the Administration. She ran the Registry extremely competently and was firm but fair. She brooked no nonsense. She had excellent interpersonal qualities and a very compassionate nature. She was liked and respected by the entire community. Her advice was invaluable and I found her support in times of crisis indispensable. Her Christian beliefs guided her actions; she was truly a force for good. The Yoruba divide people into two categories, *eniyan buruku* (bad people) and *eniyan dara dara* (good people). Bola Iluyomade was truly an *eniyan dara dara*. She retired in 2005, to my great regret—I had relied so much on her.

Mrs. E.M. Ojo, the next most senior professional in the Registry, was appointed Acting Registrar. Right from the onset, she treated me with suspicion, and, I believe, some hostility. She and Bola Iluyomade had not gotten on, because they had been in competition for years. I believe Mrs. Ojo was convinced that she had been cheated out of the position when Mrs. Iluyomade had been appointed Registrar. I suspect that her hostility to me may have been influenced by that, since she would have seen me as being close to her rival. In fact, I had made my support clear when there was a dispute over an administrative issue. I must admit that I also regarded Mrs. Ojo with some suspicion. However, she proved to be a highly competent administrator. When she was interviewed for the substantive post of Registar by a Council committee in December 2005, I pronounced that she had been carrying out her duties very capably and supported her appointment. She later told me that, when she learnt about it, she was surprised about this support. In spite of this, her guarded hostility towards me persisted until she retired a month or so before I left office. One brush that I clearly remember with her was when the University desperately needed a good Public Relations Officer. When Dele Oye informed me that Biodun Olarewaju was looking for a job after his company had been taken over, I jumped at the opportunity to employ him. He was an alumnus who I knew to be an extremely effective public relations professional, and he would be a godsend. I asked him to apply and requested the Registrar to set up an interview panel and that I wished to chair the panel. She protested, saying that the procedure was irregular. She refused to set up the panel. I told Biodun Adediran about the problem and stated that I would suspend Mrs. Ojo if she failed to carry out my directives. In the end, Biodun persuaded her to set up the panel and chair it. Biodun Olarewaju was appointed, and, as predicted, he turned out to be invaluable.

Michael Afolabi was Acting Librarian when I assumed duty. He was a hardworking man whose motives were simple—he wanted the best for his Library and he wanted the best for the University. I worked closely with him. We wanted to develop a modern, ICT-driven library. Fortunately, this was one of the components of the Carnegie Corporation project, and the Corporation recruited the Mortenson Library of the University of Illinois as our technical partner. We made some progress, but I regret to say that this was limited, mainly because of a lack of technical expertise in the Library. The Library's ICT team, led by Mrs. K. A. Jagboro, was small, and apart from Mrs. Jagboro herself, those on the team were still developing their skills through on-site and external training. This is one area where I would have liked to have seen greater progress. Anyway, back to Michael Afolabi. He was a true gentleman and we became good friends. In spite of his gentle nature, in times of crisis, he was always there to give support and advice. Indeed, he shared in the dangers on a number of occasions. One thing I could never understand was his involvement in Ekiti politics. He was deeply involved and was forever intervening to resolve the squabbles between the politicians in that State. I used to rib him about this frequently, calling him the "Chairman of the Ekiti State PDP!" He was appointed Librarian in 2001 and his appointment was renewed after his first four-year term.

Mrs. F.O. Aladekomo was the Bursar when I arrived in 1999. She was extremely good at her job, and administered the finances of the University very effectively. Like all bursars, she was rather reluctant to release funds, and those of us at the receiving end tended to be somewhat resentful of this. However, the financial survival of any organisation depends on stringent financial control. Salaries were paid on time and until she left, pensions and gratuities were also paid promptly, in spite of the serious problems that had developed with the Government's Unified Pensions Scheme. However, we did not get on too well. She was suspicious of me, and this may explain the hostility that she intermittently demonstrated. For some reason she believed that I wanted to prove that she was dishonest, possibly because she had worked with my predecessor, Wale Omole, and she saw me as antagonistic to him. This was far from the truth; I just wanted to get on with the work of administering the University. In early 2000, during a trip to Abuja, I went to the Ministry of Education to try and get a copy of the Judicial Commission's report which had just been released. Someone must have provided her with some distorted information about the visit, because when I returned, she harangued me about going from office to office looking for the report of the 1999 Visitation Panel. I had no interest in the Visitation Panel's report, but was keen to get the Judicial Panel report because of our determination to bring the 10 July murderers to justice. My denials only made the Bursar shout harder at me; this was in a meeting with other principal officers. I believe her suspicions about my intentions towards her gradually subsided over the next three years; however, our relationship remained one of tolerance. She expressed surprise when, on her retirement in April 2001, I wrote her a letter praising her achievements and her competence in administering the finances of the institution. Mrs. Lara Odeyemi, the Deputy Bursar, took over. We got on much better. However, like her predecessor, she also had the traditional finance officer's reluctance to release funds. As stated earlier, this is an essential quality of any successful bursar who wishes to ensure the financial survival of her organisation. When she was interviewed for the substantive position in February 2002, I had no hesitation in recommending her. She proved to be a very good Bursar, though somewhat acerbic towards our contractors and others who had claims on the University's finances. I occasionally had to placate individuals who had been subjected to this treatment. I also found her to be very honest; I will vouch for her any day. She was, and is, extremely loyal; she stood by me through thick and thin.

The Bursar had an extremely capable Deputy in Mrs. Ronke Akeredolu. Ronke is an excellent professional and we often called on her to deal with difficult problems. We had serious problems with the Internal Audit Department, which was functioning very poorly and where the staff were demoralised. Both problems were related to its leadership. In 2005, after a meeting with our external auditors in which they complained, yet again, that some important recommendations had not been carried out by the Department, I asked the individual concerned when he had last gone on leave. When he confirmed that he had never gone on leave, I immediately typed a memo (I used to type many of my memos personally) stating that for the sake of his health, he should proceed on all his outstanding leave immediately. This would last until well after I had left. With Lara Odeyemi's consent, we placed Ronke Akeredolu in temporary charge of the Internal Audit Department, with the task of restoring the unit to effectiveness. She achieved the task in less than three months. She organised a comprehensive staff training programme, reorganised the unit, and, on her recommendations, we promoted the qualified members of staff who had not been promoted for years. Through these measures as well as Ronke's encouragement, the morale of the staff was improved and the unit became functional once more.

Professor Wale Adebayo is a soil scientist. I put him in charge of security in the University, and he did an admirable job. Although his official title was Chairman of the Security Committee, the students called him the "Chief Security Officer." They also showed a healthy respect, indeed a fear of him. He set up the innovative "Cracker Unit" to deal with the threat of armed robbers, and this unit also served as a deterrent to secret cult activities among the students. However, in spite of the fear that the students had for the Cracker Unit, we never used it against them. Wale also organised the main security unit very effectively, and liaised with the external security agencies, including the Nigerian Police Force and the State Security Service, both of which had a great respect for him. His wife, Bisi, was a teacher. Both of them were committed members of the Baptist Church, which occupied most of their free time. Neither drank alcohol. I like a drink myself, but nevertheless we became good friends. Incidentally, he had odd eating habits, which included the fact that he never ate rice.

One other security man that I must mention is Stephen Adebanjo, known to one and all as "Banjo." He was the plain-clothed security man attached to Wale Omole, and my limited contact with him during that period suggested that he was good at his job. When I took office, everyone assumed that I would get rid of him, and, indeed, my Secretary at the time repeatedly requested me to remove him, believing that his loyalty remained with Wale Omole. My response was that he was doing his job well and that I wanted to keep him. I never regretted that decision. Banjo was absolutely loyal, and a very pleasant, unassuming and humble person. When there was some major crisis and all the regular security men had run for their lives, Banjo would remain by my side. He shared the dangers with me and was assaulted on a number of occasions. When I left office, I had hoped he would be kept on in the VC's Office, and I did speak to my successor on the matter, stating that he was absolutely loyal to the Office and to the University. However, after some time he was transferred out; he was visibly hurt by this, but soldiered on in his new post, and a second one to which he was sent some months later. Tragically, Banjo died in September 2007.

Apart from Bablo and Yemisi Obilade, the Dean and Vice-Dean of Student Affairs, there were two close friends who were important advisers on student matters. Juliet Dixon was very close to the students, and had her ear to the ground concerning their affairs. She was also a valuable adviser on matters relating to the non-academic staff unions. She was initially a secretary, but took a law degree as a mature student and subsequently joined the administrative staff. I believe her days as a mature law student facilitated the development of a deep understanding of students and their way of thinking, as well as nurturing a close relationship with students and their leaders. They truly liked her and made her the Matron of Awolowo Hall, naming her "Mama Awo." She was very close to Dorothy and I, and became one of my small circle of close friends. She did a very good job heading the Alumni Relations Department. Tragically, she became seriously ill in 2003, and died two years later. The entire community was filled with grief and I was devastated.

The second was Nick Igbokwe, a member of the Department of Physical and Health Education. My relationship with him became close over the years, and I also became close to his wife and their three delightful sons. He was a true sportsman and I made him Chairman of the Sports Council soon after my arrival, much to the discomfiture of the previous incumbent. He did a marvellous job with sports in the University. He developed a programme to increase the involvement of the University Community, particularly the students, in sports. Facilities, including basketball courts, were provided in all the halls of residence as part of the programme to decrease involvement in secret cults. He motivated and guided our sports teams so that they recorded huge successes both in the National and West African student competitions. Our contingent came second in two successive National University Games and second in the West African University Games that took place during my tenure. He was a true motivator, and the sportsmen really liked him. He knew the students inside and out, and could anticipate crises well in advance, as well as provide valuable advice when such crises occurred.

The VC's Office was run by a senior administrator, who apart from overseeing the staff in the office, acted as an administrative assistant to the VC. The first person I chose was a man who had been in the system for quite a long time and whom I had come to regard as a capable person. In fact, my knowledge of him was fairly limited; my impressions were based on what I now know to have been a very superficial appraisal. He turned out to be ineffective, but what alarmed me most was his dishonesty and disloyalty. During an industrial crisis involving the senior non-academic staff, he was reported to be openly speaking out against me, and on one occasion, as I was driving off, he said to those around him *"Were n'lo; e wo were"* ("The madman is going, see the madman.") I later found out that he had been leaking information to members of academic staff who were being processed for promotion to professorship or readership about the external assessors that I had chosen to evaluate their papers. He even gave out information on the assessors' reports. Heaven only knows what other confidences he breached. I had trusted this man and had involved him in the correspondence with the assessors. As a result of his behaviour, I drastically revised the system. I kept all the documents concerning the assessment process in a filing cabinet to which I alone had the key. I would type the nominations of assessors and take them to the Registrar personally, and I also typed the acknowledgment letters personally. The gentleman, who shall remain nameless, was replaced by Mrs. Dorothy Salami, with a personal recommendation of efficiency and integrity by the Registrar, Mrs Bola Iluyomade. What a contrast! Dorothy ran the office superbly. She is one of the best administrators I have ever met. The office was run to a very high degree of efficiency. She led the staff excellently; she was very firm with them, but also very fair. I got on excellently with her, and, above all, I trusted her. I did not need to keep looking behind my back. She also gave good advice, at least most of the time!

We got to know Professor David Ijalaye and his wife, Mrs. Joke Ijalaye, when we arrived in Ife in 1978. At that time he was the Deputy VC. He had known Dorothy's father, who, like him, was a lawyer. Uncle David is a highly respected expert in international law and is among the most renowned in his profession in Nigerian legal circles. He served as the Legal Adviser to the United Nations peace keeping mission to Somalia, and also was drafted to advise during the peace negotiations in Sierra Leone in 1999. He was one of the three who were appointed emeritus professors in 2003. Our two families have been close since 1978. Uncle David and Aunty Joke have been our greatest source of support and advice in the University since we arrived there, and this was certainly the case during my time in charge of the Hospital and the University. When serious decisions needed to be made, I would always sound him out, and when there were problems, he always had an answer. They truly cared for my family and I. Aunty Joke used to get extremely worried when things were going wrong, as they so often did. They were also an important part of my social life. If she had not seen me for a couple of weeks, Aunty Joke would complain. They occasionally visited me at home, and, of course, were present whenever I organised any event in the VC's Lodge. I loved visiting their home, a bungalow in the town. I would sit with Uncle David on the porch, drinking beer, and eating roasted guinea fowl, a constant supply of which was provided by his son, Niyi. Aunty Joke's pounded yam was a particular treat to the whole family. My son, Tony still speaks of it. I had to starve myself in advance whenever we were invited—the meal was extremely heavy, but so delicious that I would still gorge myself.

What can I say about Professor Olu Arigbabu? I met him in 1978, soon after our arrival in Ife. He is renowned for his skill as a surgeon, as well as his absolute commitment to medical practice. Patients come from all over the country to see him, and he has treated me for a number of medical problems over the years. He was loved by the entire University community because of his widely acclaimed dedication and skills in medicine. Over the years he has saved numerous lives. Most people call him by his nickname, *Oga*. Many believe that this nickname is a reflection of the numerous administrative posts that he has held over the years. In fact, the name originates from a scurrilous tale that he recited to us, concerning a platoon of soldiers and a lady of easy virtue! We went fishing together and became closer and closer. He is my closest friend. Incidentally, I taught him how to fish. Initially during our expeditions, while my two sons and I would make regular catches, he would cast repeatedly to no avail, getting more and more frustrated. I informed him that he was employing tackle that would be of more use for catching sharks and provided him with more appropriate tackle, adjusted to the right depth. He started catching fish, and did become quite an expert. However, even though he is called *Oga* (or "Master"), as far as fishing goes, I remain his master! Our social lives intertwined as our interests were more or less identical. One New Year's Eve, we both decided to stop drinking alcohol. Our resolution lasted precisely eight days. On the second Sunday of the year, we returned to his house after a fishing expedition. He sent for two bottles of Pepsi Cola. I said, "*Oga*, please, me, I want beer." His relieved response was, "Thank God!" Beer was sent for and that was the end of our resolution. As with Uncle David, I came to rely heavily on his advice and support. In earlier chapters I have described his support during various crises, both in the Hospital and the University. I relied on him, especially in times of trouble, and when things were going well, we celebrated this together. With friends like *Oga*, all problems could be overcome.

I met Dorothy when we were both medical students in the University of Ibadan. We married in 1972 after a three-year courtship. She remained my true love throughout my period of service, and my strongest source of support. She was working in Saudi Arabia when I was the Chief Medical Director in the hospital. After I finished that job and failed in my attempt to be appointed VC in 1999, we both decided to settle in England, and she took up a full time job in Watford, North London, while I planned to continue with locum consultant contracts. However, after I was appointed Acting VC in 1999 and had to change my plans, she went back to Saudi Arabia. She had not enjoyed working in Watford in any case; the facilities for her specialty, Radiology, were not up to the standard she was used to in King Saud University. Also, one of us had to earn some money! She was offered a job in one of Saudi Arabia's foremost hospitals, the National Guard Hospital in Riyadh. Thus, she was away most of the time. However, her frequent visits made up for this, when we would have a great time together—a honeymoon three times a year! When she was in Ife, she was very supportive; when she was away, I knew that I had the same unflinching support. No one can argue that the Obasanjo Administration did not record at least one major achievement, the mobile phone, and our marriage truly benefited from this. Thank you, Obasanjo!

Dorothy got caught up in student crises on two occasions. The most serious of these was the power house/Awolowo Hall incident when a miracle rescued me from a mob of students outside Awolowo Hall. She knew I had gone to deal with trouble with the students. When, after two hours I had not returned, she decided to go and look for me. She started walking in search of me with Mr. Adewale, the armed guard on duty. They first went to the Staff Club, where she found that no one had any useful information. They then proceeded to the halls of residence, arriving at Awolowo Hall to find me trapped in my vehicle. The students did not recognise her. I suspect she passed as a student. She looks much younger than I do, and much prettier! A member of academic staff recognised her there and took her home. She arrived back shortly before me. She made it a point to be with me during each Convocation period, when she truly added glamour to the occasion. Her age will not be stated here, but I assure you she still turned heads. Apart from her natural beauty, she really knows how to dress. She used to get great ovation from the students when her name was announced. I felt very proud as we arrived or left the venue, with her holding on to my arm. On those occasions, she also supervised the Convocation lunch in the VC's Lodge; she played her role as hostess very graciously. Dorothy resuscitated the Annual Children's' End-of-year Party to the great pleasure of all the children on the campus, and many outside it. On a trip to Ife in 2000, I took her to the Staff Club. The next day, I was informed that a rumour was going round that I had taken a girlfriend to the Club!

Throughout Nigeria, the term "contractor" is considered almost synonymous with corruption. There is much truth in the association. Much of the looting of our economy by politicians and Government officials ("Authority Stealing") has been done with the collusion of contractors. However, there are exceptions. I did come across a few contractors who were totally honest in their dealings with me and who demonstrated genuine professionalism in their work. The first of these is Prince E.A. Adewa, an electrical engineer whose electrical engineering firm was called "AABOWA and Sons." I got to know him when I was with the Hospital, when it became obvious to me that he ran one of the most skilled engineering companies in the country. Both in the Hospital and the University, if there was an electrical engineering job that was of a critical nature, I would be happiest if he was given the job, because I would then be absolutely confident that the work would be completed promptly; it would be of the highest quality, as well as done with absolute integrity. I used to joke with him that if I gave him a reference, many Government officials would not want to employ him, because I would state that he was both extremely capable and honest— these individuals do not want to employ honest contractors because this would prevent them from looting. There were two builders, Kayode Rotimi ("RotKay Limited") and Engineer Chris Adeloye ("Chris Adepts Limited") whom I regarded in the same way. As far as I was concerned, any carpentry work that was considered a priority would go to Tola Adesuyi and Sons, if it was at all possible. Finally, there was Engineer Bashiru Mohammed of La Mod Engineering Company, who executed our water project in Ilesa.

Over the course of this book, I have mentioned a few individuals who, in one way or the other, constituted sources of antagonism, or even worse, impediments to progress. These include the engineer that I appointed to a senior position in one of the service departments, a number of Union leaders and some student "leaders," who would be better described as "misleaders." There are a few more that need to be mentioned. Otas Ukponmwan has always been in the forefront of the activities of ASUU, and was Chairman of the local branch in 1999 and 2000. We did not get on well. That in itself would not have been a major problem; I did not get on well with a number of other people but this did not prevent us from working together. However, his antagonism went beyond that. He went out of his way to criticise and antagonise me, and eventually, developed a persecution "complex" towards me and even about those who were close to me. There were frequent accusations of persecution. One evening, he went over to *Oga* Arigbabu's house (he lived next door to him at the time) in a state of severe agitation. He stated that he had been followed home by the Crackers and that they had been instructed by me to kill him. In fact, the Cracker vehicle had followed his car on the way to dropping off a guard at *Oga* Arigbabu's house. *Oga* managed to calm him down and opened a bottle of whiskey. After consuming a major part of the bottle, *Oga* informed him that I was the one who had given him the drink on my return from a trip abroad. He appeared unconcerned by this announcement, drank a substantial amount of the drink and was eventually escorted, staggering, to his house by the Cracker who was guarding *Oga*'s house. On another occasion, he created a major fuss when I refused to accept a drink from him in the Staff Club. He had sent over a beer to me where I was sitting and I sent it back, stating that I had not asked for it. I felt that the action was insulting; if he wanted to buy me a beer, he should have had the courtesy to ask me first. He exploded, and for days afterwards he went round the campus loudly complaining that I had refused to accept the beer from him. The most hilarious event occured when I once went into the Staff Club toilet to find him inside. He immediately ran out, loudly complaining that I had come to attack him in the toilet! After I left office, we became reasonably cordial. Tragically, Otas died recently. May his soul rest in peace.

In the initial period of my service as VC, secret cult activity constituted the major antisocial problem. The problem was largely contained within the first year, though it was not completely eliminated. However, what little activity there was remained largely underground. Two other major problems were rampant—sexual assault and harassment and cheating at examinations. Early on at least, there was a general attitude among both male staff and male students that the exploitation of women was socially acceptable, and that, indeed, this was the norm. Sexual harassment was common as a result, and there were cases of male members of academic staff using their power over female undergraduates to seduce them. This "power" they had was merely the superior position of a teacher to his student. However, there were also frequent cases of male academic staff using the threat of examination failure or the "reward" of advantageous marks to commit what can only be described as rape. Of course, in some cases the girls themselves sought relationships with lecturers because of the attraction of befriending such a "superior" being. I know of occasions when girls actually deliberately used sex to get passes or good marks. However, most of the time the coercion came from the lecturer. I inherited one particularly bad case involving the Faculty of Social Sciences, but those involved managed to get away with it through a successful cover-up. There were other cases thereafter, but in most cases we could not pin the perpetrators down because they used a combination of bribery and threats to ensure that the victims or witnesses did not come forward. Incidentally, I never came across any case of sexual harassment of males by females; however, that does not mean that this did not occasionally occur.

In February 2001, I received a letter from a parent complaining that his daughter had allegedly been kidnapped and held for some hours in a lecturer's house. That lecturer seemed to have developed some notoriety already. Shortly before I received the complaint, the lecturer had reported that he had emerged from his flat one morning to find that his Volkswagen car had been lifted up onto the stairs! Presumably this was the work of some students. The parent attached a detailed report of the incident provided by the victim. This was a first-year student who had been offered a lift by the lecturer outside their Faculty. He had offered to take her to her residence. Instead, he drove her to his flat and held her there overnight. I immediately phoned the complainant and promised immediate action. A panel was set up and the panel's report confirmed the incident. In accordance with the University's laws, the matter was reported to the Appointments and Promotions Committee and then to Council. A joint committee of Council and Senate took up the case and found he had behaved inappropriately. Council, after consultation with the University Senate, dismissed him. He went to court and the case is still sub judice.

Rape, at least in its narrower sense of violent sexual assault, was much more frequently committed by male against female students. These included horrific episodes of multiple rape by groups of male students. Most of the cases occurred at night and I often received calls from the Health Centre concerning them. I always responded to these calls, first because I felt immediate counselling and support was required and also because I needed to convince the victims to give evidence so that we could bring the perpetrators to book. These young victims were understandably reluctant to give evidence and submit to the intimate medical examinations required to collect the evidence. They often felt ashamed, and also afraid of revenge from the perpetrators. I referred all the cases to an organisation called Women Against Rape, Sexual Abuse and Harassment (WARSHE) for longer term counselling of the victims. That organisation also gave support to the victims during the distressing course of the investigations of these cases, and the disciplinary actions that followed. I dealt very firmly with the perpetrators; once the investigation confirmed that the rape had taken place, they would be immediately expelled. Some cases were also reported to the police, but invariably no criminal prosecution occurred. WARSHE proved an invaluable ally in dealing with cases of sexual harassment and assault. They were even more important in the efforts of the University to educate and orientate female students about their rights. They organised a number of programmes on this, and also took part in the annual orientation programme for new students. The organisation was led by Yemisi Obilade, who I appointed the Vice-Dean of Student Affairs, as well as an equally committed colleague from the same faculty (Education), Dr. Toyin Fasina.

Cheating at examinations was rampant in the University, and, with the support of the University Senate, I decided to deal firmly with the problem. Students used a variety of methods to cheat. Most commonly, they would come to the examination hall with "microchips," pieces of tightly rolled up paper on which important points were inscribed in tiny handwriting. Some students would pay others to take examinations for them. From time to time, examiners would report identical scripts from two students. There were cases of students breaking into lecturers' offices to steal copies of examination questions or to copy them. Leakage of examination papers occurred in a number of other ways. Clerical officers, typists, or messengers might retain copies of question papers during the preparation or duplication of examination papers and, occasionally, lecturers leaked examination questions to their girlfriends. Of course, lecturers could employ much more subtle means of assisting individuals, for the reward of sex or money, by informing students of the specific subjects that were to appear on the examination paper and by over-generous awards of marks. This latter method was extremely difficult to detect.

We were able to detect and prosecute some cases of the changes of marks by lecturers, but I suspect that in most cases, they went undetected. Perhaps the most elaborate examination fraud was the case of the "Magic Pencils." Some students stole a copy of a multiple choice paper in anatomy, and transcribed the correct answers onto slips of paper which were tightly wrapped around the ends of the "magic pencils" and sold to a substantial number of medical students. I expelled more than 20 students over that episode. Cases of examination malpractice were investigated by three committees that were responsible for cases from different faculties. Their recommendations would be sent to me. Initially, I went along with their recommendations, which were usually for suspensions from the University. In 2003, I decided, with the support of the University Senate, to introduce a harsher punishment—expulsion. I issued a release to this effect and instituted this harsher punishment. Expelled students had a right of appeal to the Governing Council, and initially, the Council tended to commute the expulsions to terms of suspension. However, after a year, I was able to convince the Council to uphold the harsher punishments. The frequency of examination malpractice was reduced drastically thereafter. One case caused me great distress, which was when I had to expel the son of a friend.

Each year, up to 100,000 young people would apply to "Great Ife," and up to half of those would achieve the University's minimum entry requirement of 200 in the University

Matriculation Examination plus five School Certificate credits. Only about 5,000 would be admitted. Unscrupulous people, both staff and students, would take advantage of the desperation of candidates and their parents to defraud them through promises of admission. Up to ₦100,000 or more would change hands. In most cases, the prospective student would arrive, armed with forged admission documents, only to be turned away. We caught a number of these fraudsters, usually when the enraged victims of these confidence tricks reported cases. The culprits were invariably dismissed. However, I know that there were some admission rackets that were virtually institutionalised, with those charged with the responsibility for the admissions in faculties being involved. These were much more difficult to detect because the candidates got in and thus did not complain. A similar and very widespread racket was the selling of bed spaces in the halls of residence. Less than one-third of the students were entitled to bed spaces. It was common practice for a student to sell his bed space for which a charge of ₦2590 was made by the University for between ₦25,000 and ₦30,000. Yet, when the charge of ₦2,500 for hostel maintenance was introduced, the students rioted!

One of the most disgraceful features of the University's academic functions during my period as VC was the failure to process examination results. I have already described how results were withheld as a tool in the Union's fight with me. However, from my first Senate meeting to the last, it was clear that, even during "peacetime," results were not being processed on schedule. A large backlog of results had accumulated during the 1990s. Students normally need their results to register for each semester, and, indeed, some courses were prerequisites to subsequent courses. The result was chaos. Students would continue with their studies, not knowing whether they were actually qualified to be in their year of study or whether they were qualified for the courses they were currently taking. The matter reached tragic proportions when in, January 2002, a large number of students were asked to withdraw after the results from two and three years back were finally processed.

I am surprised that these students did not take us to court. The Deans had to hold a substantial number of special meetings, backed up by a combination of pleas and threats from the Administration, to clear the backlog. The two successive Deputy VCs (Administration), Wale Akinsola and Biodun Adediran, drove the process. We did clear most of it, but lost ground again during the protracted confrontation with ASUU. After that crisis, we had to go through the whole rigmarole again; however, we had cleared most of the results by the time I left.

The account of how the "Cracker Unit" was established has earlier been given. There is no doubt that this unit was instrumental in restoring security to the University. However, there were some drawbacks to their activities, two of them extremely serious. On one occasion a teacher in the Staff School was accidentally shot at a road block while operating an illegal taxi service. He was in hospital for quite a long time and almost lost his left leg. On 6 August 2002, I heard over the walkie-talkie system that there was an emergency situation at the Infinite Grace Supermarket within the Staff Quarters. I drove there to be confronted with a horrific scene. Wale Adebayo joined me there soon afterwards. A young man was lying on the ground dead, with his skull blown out by a shotgun wound. A number of Crackers were there, and their leader, Mr. Hassan, was spattered with blood and brains. A hysterical young lady was screaming that the Crackers had killed her fiancé. The dead man was Cyriacus Ugonna Ekeh, a final- year student of Geology. He had gone to the cybercafe attached to the supermarket and then got into a shouting match with the staff over his bill. He was said to have used threatening language. The manager of the supermarket had telephoned the security control room, allegedly saying that an armed robbery attack was in progress. The Crackers had rushed to the scene and, during a confrontation with Ugonna, a shot had been fired. I conferred with Wale and Mr. Hassan. However, our course of action was straightforward. We sent for the Police, who, of course, immediately arrested the Cracker whose gun had been fired. I then proceeded to the Students' Union building with Wale to inform the student leaders of the incident. We were already in the middle of a student crisis, and the situation was made even thornier by this. The students immediately called a congress in the amphitheatre and I had to go and address them. It was a very difficult time; the student leaders, headed by Olawoyin, capitalised on the episode to condemn the University's security services and the Crackers in particular. I was personally abused. I just had to stand there taking it; all I could say was how grief-stricken I was. We later had a meeting with the student leaders and senior academic staff and agreed to set up an enquiry into the security system. I must say that the panel did not yield any really useful recommendations. However, we did institute additional training for the Cracker Unit.

Worse was to come; we had to face Ugonna's relatives. A member of the electrical staff, Desmond Njoku, who was from Ugonna's town, Ngor Okpala, offered to travel there to inform the relatives. Professor C.U. Manus, also from that area, offered practical advice and volunteered to participate in the discussions with the family. I must mention here that not everyone was so helpful. There was a very senior member of the Department of Geology who came from Ngor Okpala and who would have been a great source of assistance with the relatives of the victim. He bluntly refused to help, and I later learnt that he was the source of a claim by some members of the community that the University was anti-Ibo, and a Yoruba would never have been "murdered" in that manner. The family arrived a week after the killing. I believe we were able to convince them of our deep regret and grief over Ugonna's death. Professor Manus and Mr. Njoku conducted most of the discussion, or, should I say, negotiations. We agreed on compensation for the family. We also agreed that the University would make all the funeral arrangements and pay all costs of their travel, and I would personally lead a delegation to the funeral. I was joined by Professor C.O. Umoru, the Dean of the Faculty of Science, for the trip. We spent the night in Owerri and travelled to Ngor Okpala on the morning of the funeral. We arrived at about 9am and proceeded to the family home, where we were confronted by an angry relative asking why we had killed their son. There were others showing hostility, but a senior member of the community took us to his home and reassured us of our safety. The Director of the State Security Service in Osogbo had also arranged for a member of that service from Imo State to be present in case there was any danger to us. Fortunately, his services were not required, and in fact, after the initial hostility, we were treated fairly well. Throughout the funeral, I was in a daze. I do recall much grief and tears from the entire community as Ugonna was buried.

One of the major causes that ASUU took up was the crisis in the University of Ilorin. The Ilorin branch of the Union was particularly militant; indeed only the Ife branch surpassed it in this respect. When ASUU declared strike action in 2001, the Ilorin branch, which was already in dispute with the administration of the University, joined in immediately. The relationship of the members of the branch with the VC there was particularly bad; thus the University's administration took the matter as a personal affront, and so did its Governing Council. The Council gave an ultimatum for the lecturers to go back to work, and an attendance register was opened, which many of the lecturers signed. However, the more militant of them refused to go back to work or sign the register. The Governing Council then ordered them to be sacked. Letters of dismissal were issued and the lecturers ordered to vacate their quarters overnight. The VC backed up this order by sending security men and thugs to evict them. Those who did not go were forcibly removed along with their wives and children and their belongings thrown out onto the road.

The lecturers went to court and obtained an injunction. However, the University refused to obey the court order. When a bailiff was sent to deliver the court order, he was beaten up. ASUU's next national strike action included the perceived injustice to these unfortunate lecturers and their families as the major issue. The President even got involved and backed the Ilorin Governing Council's action. There was a prolonged stalemate.

In late 2002, the Committee of Vice-Chancellors (CVC) decided to intervene. It set up a team of four Vice-Chancellors to visit the University, ascertain the facts and provide recommendations for a solution. The members of the team were to meet in Ilorin. In the event only two of us showed up, the VC of the University of Maiduguri and I. I guess the other two suspected that they might be in for trouble. The two of us met with the VC, Professor Oba Abdulraheem. He gave a story of protracted indiscipline and disruption by those who had been sacked. He introduced us to a purported new Ilorin branch of ASUU. This was a group of obviously cowed individuals who asserted that they were working actively with the VC and that the lecturers that had been dismissed were a group of vagabonds and saboteurs. However, we knew that this new group was not recognised by the national body of ASUU, which continued to insist that the original executive, all of whom had been sacked, was the legitimate executive.

We arranged to meet the ASUU members that had been sacked. The meeting was arranged for 9am the next day at a hotel in the town. On arrival we found the dismissed lecturers outside the gates of the hotel, which had been locked. The Police had issued a directive to the manager that the meeting should not be allowed to take place there. They had found another hotel where the meeting could take place and we moved there. I almost wept when they described what had happened to them. They had been on a legitimate strike action, well within their rights, and had been dismissed and thrown out of their homes with their families. None of them had even been given so much as a query before they were sacked.

What became immediately obvious, even from the VC's evidence, was that in dismissing the lecturers, the laws of the nation had been trampled upon. The enabling law of the University of Ilorin, which is one of the laws of the Federation of Nigeria, lays down a procedure for the discipline of members of academic staff. The procedure involves informing the individual concerned of the offence(s) for which he is charged and allowing him to defend himself against the allegations before a joint committee of the Governing Council and the University Senate. None of this was done; they were just dismissed outright by the Council. The Obasanjo Government backed the Governing Council's actions.

XXII

End of Another Term

M y term was due to end on 5 May 2006. Those last few months were very busy for me. I spent a lot of time on the Renovation Project and on other aspects of University Advancement.

As the date of my exit was approaching, the Pro-Chancellor appointed Biodun Adediran to chair a committee to organise a send-off. When he approached me, I stated very firmly that I did not want a send-off and wished to leave quietly. I really did not want any fuss, and also, I felt that many of those who would attend such an event did not have much regard for me; indeed, some of them hated my guts. I did participate in a small send-off in the office, at which Mrs. Ojo, my secretary of many years, was to have her retirement celebrated. A number of departments invited me round and presented me with gifts, often turning these into mini send-offs. I thought I had avoided any fuss, but my friends insisted on a celebration. They believed that whatever had been achieved during my term was worth celebrating; more importantly, they wanted to celebrate my physical survival as well as surviving in office to the end of my term. As I have mentioned earlier, of my seven predecessors, only three had completed their terms; the others had been unceremoniously removed from office. I agreed to a small get-together in the VC's Lodge on 6 May. I had thought the event would comprise a small gathering of close friends over a few bottles of beer and wine, and, possibly, some suya. I started getting worried when a canopy arrived at the lodge. By the evening of the event, it was obvious that this was to be no small gathering but a very elaborate affair; however, by then it was too late. It was a truly memorable evening. It started with an hour of praise worship, followed by a delicious dinner involving a very varied menu. There were speeches, by individuals who obviously meant what they said. We danced to a live band well into the night. I was truly moved. My friends had spent a huge sum on the send-off out of their love for me. Every person who attended truly had a high regard for me, and was clearly delighted that I was completing my term of office after a very torrid seven years. The only sad thing was that Peter, Nick and Ify Igbokwe's youngest child, was ill in hospital, so they could not attend the party. I am happy to record that the little boy recovered fully.

I was packed and ready to go. The next morning, albeit with hangovers, my friends, the faithful Grace and the two stewards, Lawrence and Raji, gathered round and saw me off. I drove to the airport and travelled to London that night. So ended my adventure of seven turbulent years.

I constantly look back over the seven eventful years, trying to appraise the achievements and the failures, and to determine whether the balance was positive or negative. Of course, that final judgment would be impossible for me. No person can truly appraise himself; only objective observers can do so. And, since so many of the observers during the period were actively, and even emotionally, involved, most of them also cannot make an objective assessment. Only posterity can make a truly objective appraisal. I do know that there were some major achievements, and I know also that there were some failures.

I was able to show that, even in Nigeria, it is possible to hold a position of responsibility without abusing it, and, in particular, without enriching yourself. I believe my position in this respect, of total integrity with the University's finances, did influence a substantial number of the staff, and probably also the students. People respond to their leaders, and, they try to emulate them. There were, of course, exceptions; examples of these have been given earlier. The contractors and suppliers also responded positively to this position. The reality of present-day Nigeria is that contractors have to tailor their approach to those they deal with. If they know that they have to give bribes, which, of course, means that they have to inflate prices, then they will. But the converse also applies. Between 1999 and 2006, they knew they did not have to "give" to get a contract or to get a payment approved or processed. The result was that the University benefited through lower prices and higher standards of performance.

I hope I was able to motivate some of the academic staff. I know that, in spite of the serious conflict over "no work, no pay," some at least did acknowledge my values, as well as my desire for high academic standards. I tried, and I hope, succeeded in motivating non-academic staff by demonstrating how important their jobs were. I know that I did leave a lasting impression on the majority of the students. While it is true that the student leaders were in constant conflict with me for much of the time, these student leaders constituted only a small minority of the student body. The vast majority of the students had a high regard for me. I was very visible to them; some of the academic staff accused me of being too accessible. The students knew I was committed to their welfare. I hope my stand on corruption also filtered down to them. Wherever I go in the country and outside it, young (and old) alumni come up to me and proudly say "Sir, I was at Ife." I always encourage them to continue projecting a good image of the institution, to support the University and to join the Alumni Association.

The development of Advancement activities, begun under my predecessor, really took off during my term. I am really proud of our breakthrough in achieving the first Carnegie Corporation grant and getting it renewed, against competition from many other institutions. The University Community was extremely resistant to the idea of fundraising; by the time I left, the essential nature of University Advancement was widely accepted.

The University became a much safer place. The secret cult menace was largely overcome; in this, the students played an indispensable role. The Cracker Unit kept us safe from armed robbers and also was a major deterrent on the operation of secret cults; however, we never used the Crackers against students. The OAU Campus is now one of the safest places in Nigeria.

The outcomes on staff and students unions were mixed. NASU and SSANU were dealt with very firmly in 2000 and 2001, and their excesses during industrial actions ceased. The Students' Union certainly constituted a major problem throughout the period, but we were able to stand up to them. Thus, in spite of their violent antagonism, we were able to introduce the new charges that made such a great difference to the conditions in which they lived and the quality of our academic programmes. The conflict with ASUU was a different matter—the Union dealt with me! They won hands down.

In spite of the very limited funding available, we did get a substantial number of new projects done. The Central Science Laboratory, initiated by my predecessor, Wale Omole, is one of the most important. This concept has been copied by many other universities in West Africa. The OAU International School has made a great difference to the University Community. The Link Road with the Teaching Hospital, apart from its practical value to staff and students commuting between the two institutions, has saved many lives. Although we built twelve new hostel blocks, these provided only a small proportion of the bed spaces required. Clearly, private sector investment in student hostel accommodation is the only viable solution. Modest beginnings were recorded in this area during my term and that of my predecessor; I am glad that this is now attracting more investors.

The Centre for Industrial Research and Development truly achieved its mandate and potential under the leadership of Funmi Togonu-Bickersteth. The Institute of Agricultural Research and

Training in Ibadan became one of the few research institutions in the country that were actually performing; in the face of dwindling funding from the government, it developed into a very strong research institute under the innovative leadership of Professor J.O. Ojo-Atere and then Professor Anthony Adebowale. Gender equity became a reality in the institution, driven by the influence (and the funds) of the Carnegie Corporation and midwifed by the Center for Gender and Social Policy Studies. Women and girls in OAU were truly liberated. Cultural Studies returned to the forefront. I am proud of our success in once more bringing into prominence one of the four major objectives of the University's founding fathers—the promotion and study of African Cultures. It is a pity that the second edition of the resuscitated Ife International Festival of Arts and Culture had to be postponed because of the political climate in the country. However, Wole Soyinka kept his promise to direct this when it was successfully organised in 2008. The Center for Distance Learning, which took off so strongly, will play a key role in the future of the University.

The natural environment of the campus remained as beautiful as ever, in spite of the constraints. The Reforestation Project has made a major difference and its effects will continue to increase as the years go on. I am very sad that the achievements of Sina Aderibigbe in restoring the Teaching and Research Farm were not built on by his successors as deans. Indeed, the farm was beginning to look more and more like a barren desert. However, on a visit to Ife in 2010, I was delighted to see that the Farm was once more back to life; all it takes is a good leader.

What about academics? Our students continued to excel nationally. Our graduates were in great demand by the multinationals. On successive years, our graduates won the Star Prize at the Nigerian Law School's examinations. We were the first to introduce entrepreneurship programmes, but even before that our graduates were renowned for not only being highly employable but also of being able to create their own employment. Graduates of the University are leading the way in their respective professions all over the world. The National

Universities Commission declared OAU as the leading research institution in the country when they appraised the University System in 2004. I was in sticking to our guns in the face of an increasingly untenable position thus prolonging the strike. And, of course, it is not just about academics; our students were in the forefront in sports.

I regret to admit that the failings are also well represented in this account. I made some faulty appointments, especially that of the Engineer whose escapades have been described.

Some observers believe that the major violent confrontations, one with NASU and several others with the Students' Union would perhaps not have reached such violent proportions if I had handled them differently. There is one other important issue—it is my firm belief that any Vice-Chancellor who runs away from his students would not have their respect and has no business being Vice-Chancellor. On the 3 November, 2004, if I had not gone to my office, the students would have come to the Vice-Chancellor's Lodge and invaded it. I do have one major regret—the student, Olalekan Laketu, would have been alive today if I had retreated on 3 November 2004. I will always have that young man's death on my conscience.

However, the major failing was in my dealings with ASUU. The University was closed for a total of 22 months during my seven years in office. This was more than in any other university during that period. The greatest proportion of these lost months was the result of the confrontation by ASUU over the "two steps" issue and the subsequent local action over the issue of the withheld salaries. On reflection, I must accept the blame for the latter. I made two major errors in dealing with the problem. I should have realised that ASUU had a much stronger resolve than SSANU and NASU. They were truly determined; they believed in their cause. The first error was in underestimating that resolve. The second was in. Once the salaries had been stopped, I should never have gone back on it. Instead, I compounded the first error with the second. However, I must state here and now that I believe in the principle of "No work, No pay". If unions believe in a cause, then they should have the courage of their convictions. In almost all countries, unions ensure that they have built up enough financial resources to implement "strike pay" when they bring their members out on strike. The only way to put an end to the incessant strike actions, many of them irresponsible ones, in our country is to implement this internationally accepted convention. The conflict was between ASUU and the Government, and latterly between ASUU and the University Administration; actually, many saw it as a conflict between ASUU and Roger Makanjuola. The ultimate losers were our students. I have publicly apologised to our students. May they forgive us...

XXIII

Postscript–Return to Ife

I love the Ife Campus. After my departure as Vice-Chancellor, I spent the next year in England, where I was reunited once more with my family. Once more, I took up locum consultant appointments and thoroughly enjoyed the work. It was a peaceful and enjoyable respite, but I loved Ife, and had promised to return. I did so in January 2007. Kwashi Ako-Nai had allocated a professorial house to me in a quiet close, and it had been refurbished and furnished. I was very happy there. I resumed my work as a teacher and a consultant in the hospital and was fulfilled. I was the first VC to return to the University after his term ended and I was welcomed back by every member of the Community; well, almost everybody. Wherever I went on the Campus I was received and treated with a great deal of courtesy and consideration. I felt I truly belonged. Once, when I blundered into the middle of a student demonstration, I was greeted with delighted shouts of "Roja, Roja, Roja;" The weekends were great spending Friday and Saturday evenings in the Staff Club with my friends; yes, the same friends who had been with me during my turbulent seven years in charge. There was good fishing in the reservoirs on Sundays and we transferred the Sunday afternoon parties that we had previously held in the VC's Lodge to my new house. Life was good and still is.

I love Great Ife.

Index